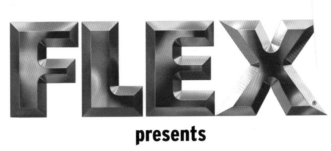

FLEX

presents

HUGE

A Complete Workout Regimen from Bodybuilding's Superstars

"Strive for excellence, exceed yourself, love your friends, speak the truth, practice fidelity, and honor your father and mother. These principles will help you master yourself, make you strong, give you hope and put you on the path to greatness."

Joe Weider

— Joe Weider, Trainer of Champions Since 1936

Dear Reader,
Since its inception in 1983, FLEX magazine has been the bible of bodybuilding and the number one source for training and nutrition information. Now we've created HUGE, a book-length compendium of all the bodybuilding knowledge we've accumulated over the years. This book is based on articles and information in FLEX magazine that you have enjoyed and learned from. We know you'll love HUGE as much as you love FLEX.

— The Editors of FLEX

ACKNOWLEDGMENTS

Photos by Bob Gardner, John Kelly, Chris Lund, Robert Reiff and Art Zeller. Illustrations by Stuart Weiss. Project Editor is Jeanine Detz. Project Art Director is Kimberly Richey. FLEX Editor-in-Chief is Peter McGough. Creative Director is Chris Hobrecker. Editor is Michael Berg. Managing Editor is Vicki Baker. Senior Art Director is Kiwon Ballman. Art Director is Kimberly Mitru Ludeke. Production Manager is Kathy Conrad. Director of Rights and Permissions is Fiona Maynard. Vice President, Global Licensing and Product Development is Jonathan Bigham. Founding Chairman is Joe Weider. Chairman, President, CEO is David Pecker.

ISBN 978-1-57243-974-0

Printed in China.

CONTENTS

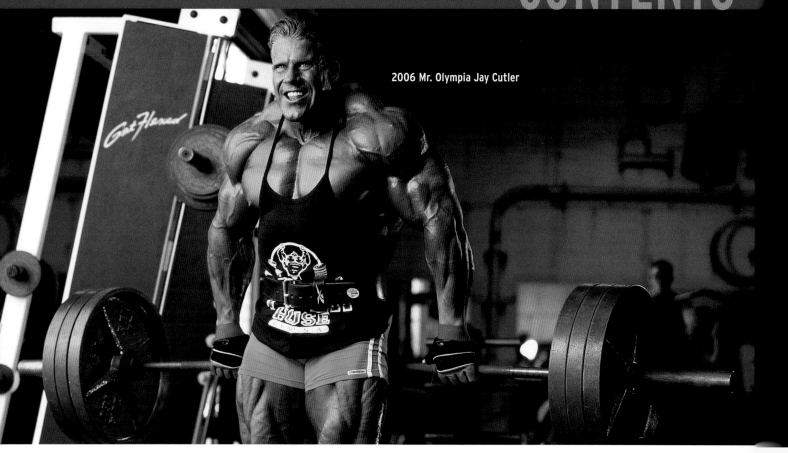

2006 Mr. Olympia Jay Cutler

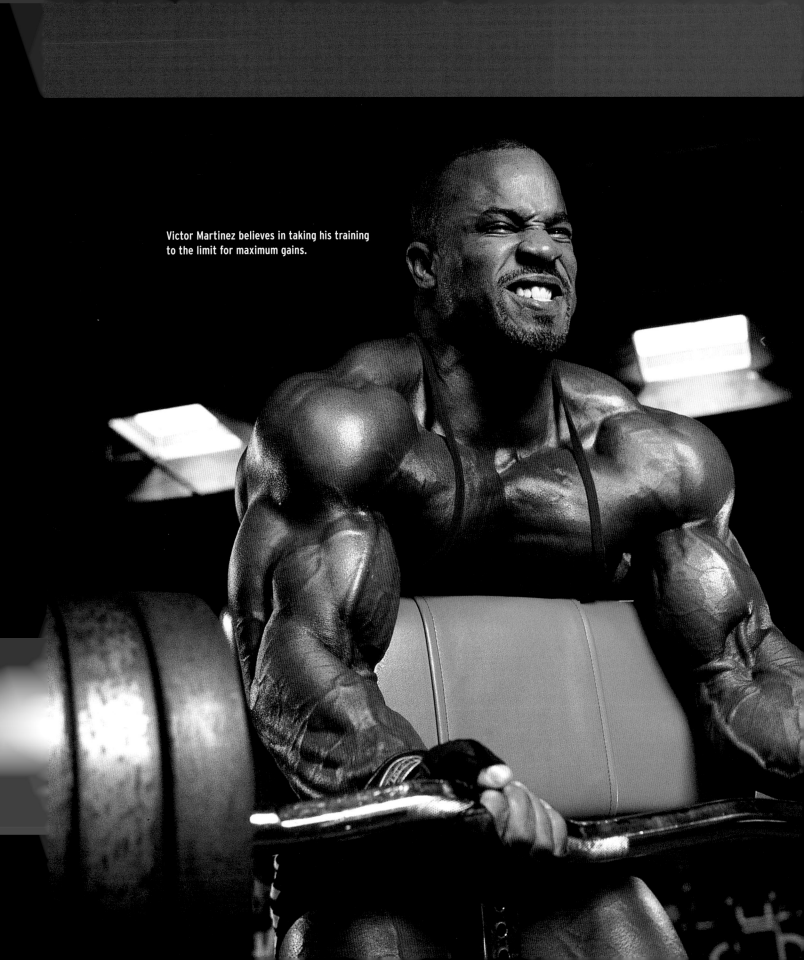

Victor Martinez believes in taking his training to the limit for maximum gains.

CONTENTS

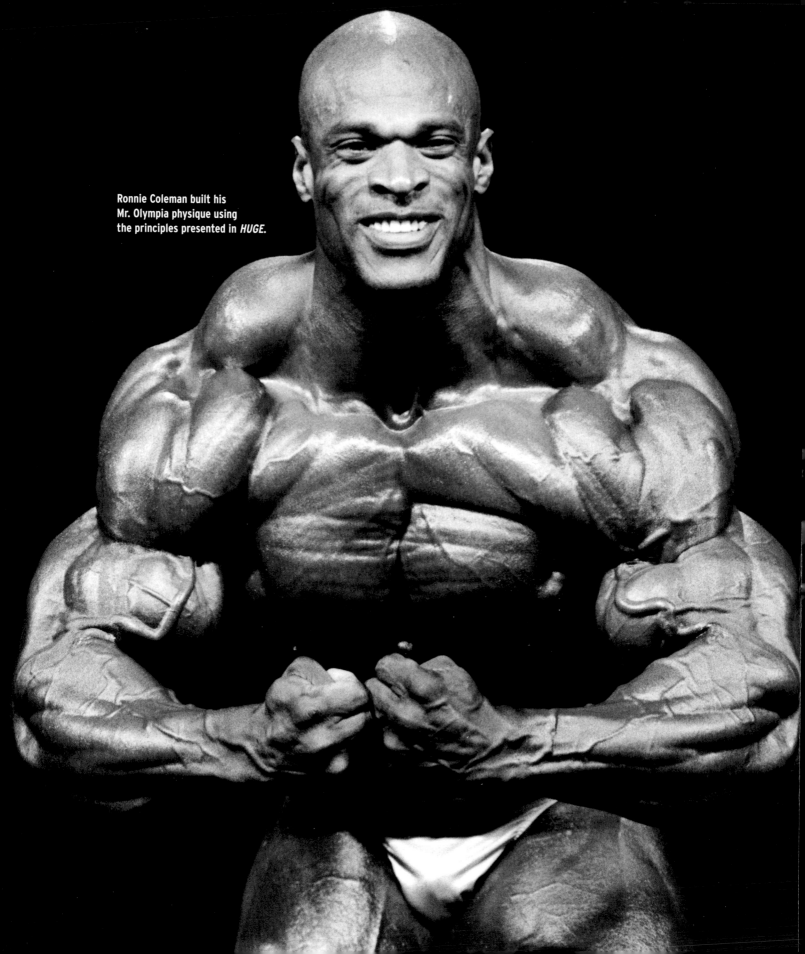

Ronnie Coleman built his Mr. Olympia physique using the principles presented in *HUGE*.

Your Introduction
TO BIGNESS

You hold in your hands the ultimate guide to Bigness. Whether you're a rank beginner or a seasoned veteran, *HUGE* is your passport to new and improved levels of muscularity.

With its cutting-edge information on training, nutrition, supplementation and the science of changing body composition, *FLEX* magazine has long been recognized as the bible of bodybuilding. Now, we've done something we've never done before: We've published a book, distilling all this information into an easy-to-follow program for muscle growth.

You will benefit from our unbridled reservoir of knowledge with instruction on exercises, training phases, nutrition, recovery and supplementation. No matter who you are or what your level of bodybuilding experience, you can make the gains you've always wanted with *HUGE*.

GETTING STARTED

So, how can one book be right for all bodybuilders? The answer to that question is contained within these pages. If you're a first-time bodybuilder, or one who hasn't trained for some time, you'll want to pay particular attention to the first section of the book, "Welcome to Bodybuilding." More experienced trainers should also read this section but may be able to skip "The First Four Weeks" training section, and go straight into the 13-week "Mass Attack" program. The beginners' four-week training cycle is designed to allow your muscles and body to accommodate to the rigors of training for the first time or after a long period of inactivity. Once

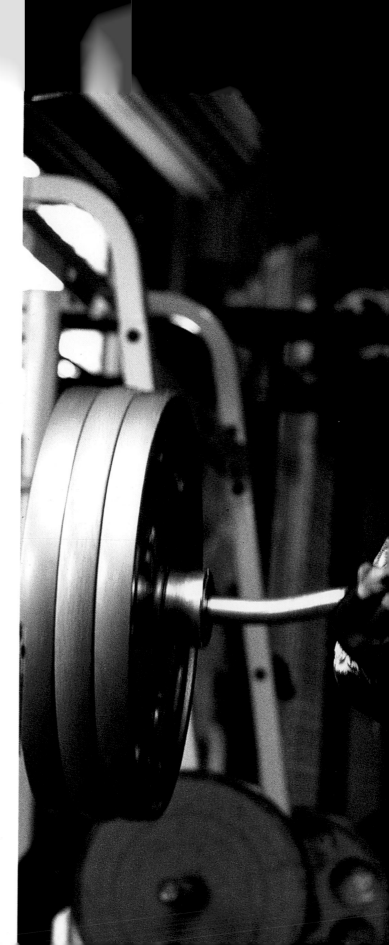

your body has made this adaptation, you'll be ready for our next phase: "Mass Attack."

Can you build a world-class physique? Maybe. Maybe not. It depends on your genetics and, more importantly, on your dedication. One thing we can promise you, though, is that if you are a beginning bodybuilder following the program in this book, you will make better gains in your first year — particularly if you're young — than at any other time in your bodybuilding endeavors. Even if you do have experience, you may be surprised by how much success you'll have when you religiously follow the instruction provided in this book.

All professional bodybuilders know they can only make a certain amount of improvement in a given length of time. Ask a pro such as Jay Cutler or Ronnie Coleman what his goal is for the next year, and he'll tell you he wants to sharpen up a couple bodyparts and add a few pounds of mass. These goals

Plan ahead, work with your body and begin to learn what works for you and how to implement these strategies.

may seem fairly modest — and they are — but the important thing is that they are attainable. Ronnie and Jay have had goals like this for years; so, when you string together a decade or more of goals and successful completion, you can see how these pros built their world-class physiques.

GROWTH CYCLES

Once you start training, your initial gains will be impressive. Like the pros, though, you will eventually start to plateau as you take your physique as far as you can with your initial program. That's where *HUGE* comes in. We show you how to take your training to the next level, whatever level you start from. It's important to recognize the cyclical nature of bodybuilding growth. The fastest route to perfecting your physique is not in charging straight ahead and training to the point of exhaustion and over-stimulation. Rather, the best philosophy is to plan ahead, a few months at a time, work with your body and begin to learn what works for you and how to implement these strategies.

YOUR INTRODUCTION TO BIGNESS

Chris Cormier started training as a teenager to build his championship physique.

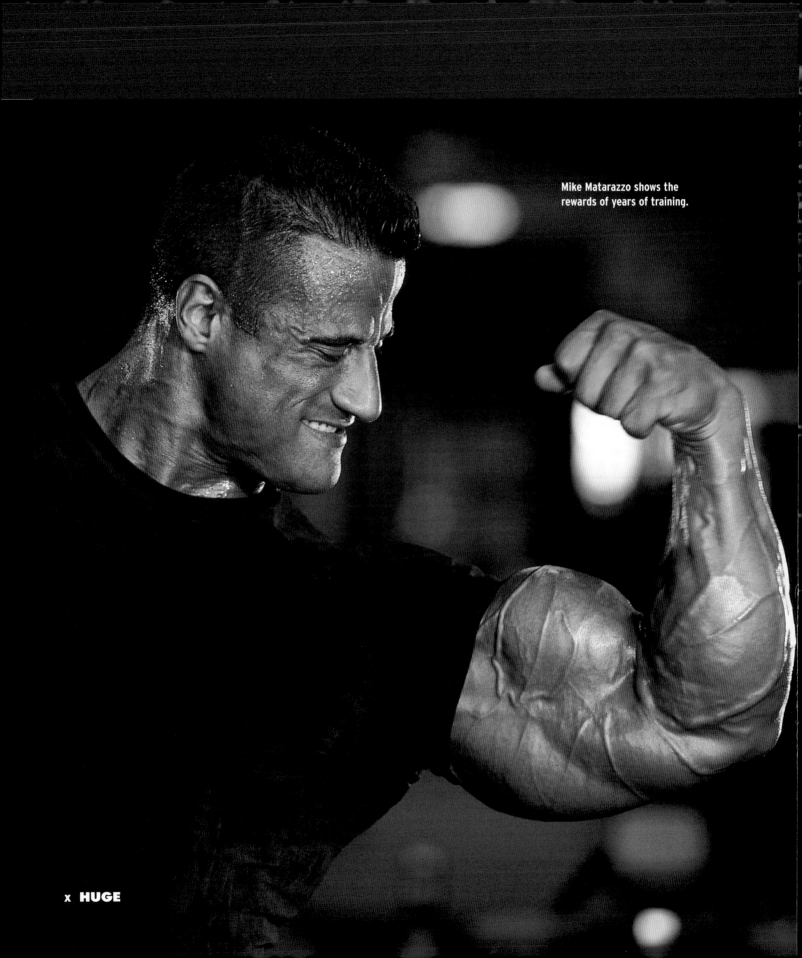

Mike Matarazzo shows the rewards of years of training.

Throughout the book, we provide different workout strategies, including a beginning phase ("The First Four Weeks"), a muscle-building regimen ("Mass Attack"), a 13-week power surge ("Three-Month Power Program"), a change-up routine to provide variety ("The Next Step") and a final 13-week cutting phase ("Rip It Up") which will help you take all the muscle you've added and display it to its best advantage. We're giving you over a year's worth of programs and training cycles, and we carefully explain the rationale for each.

In addition, *HUGE* provides all you need to know about basic bodybuilding nutrition and supplementation to put on the quality pounds of muscle you're seeking. One mistake many bodybuilders make is to devote all their efforts to training at the expense of nutrition. *HUGE* explains the need for increasing calories for growth, and the nutritional shifts you need to make to reduce bodyfat while maintaining your hard-earned muscle. Emphasize nutrition at the same time that you emphasize a new training regimen, and your gains will go through the roof. The bottom line is that bodybuilding-friendly nutrition will support and influence your gym efforts, and accelerate muscle growth.

We also give you advanced information on training technique — Chapter Four, "Perfect Form," explains how to perform the ideal rep, and it is the essence of the *FLEX* bodybuilding philosophy. Plus, we tell you how to get inspired and stay motivated, how to work out for your bodytype, how to use advanced training techniques and how to include shock tactics for overcoming training plateaus. In short, we give you everything you need to know for bodybuilding success.

KEYS TO SUCCESS:
EXPERIENCE AND INSPIRATION

As you go through the workout phases, keep in mind that all bodies are different, and each responds differently to various types of muscular stimulation. Part of your job is to pay attention to what works best for you. After you complete the first year of this program, you'll want to rebuild your workout using the concepts you've learned for the next year's plan. Our final chapter, "Now It's Up To You," explains how you can take your future bodybuilding program into your own hands.

Of course, you're going to want to continue to read *FLEX* magazine, and continue to refer to this book. No matter how well you know the subject matter, every time you return to

FLEX you'll find inspiration. Flip through the book and look at the pros in action. These guys train hard and *FLEX* photographer Chris Lund and others dynamically capture all their blood, sweat and muscles. You'll find similar images in each issue of *FLEX* magazine.

So, start reading the book, keep reading the magazine and get started on your path to physique greatness. *FLEX* will change your life. We promise.

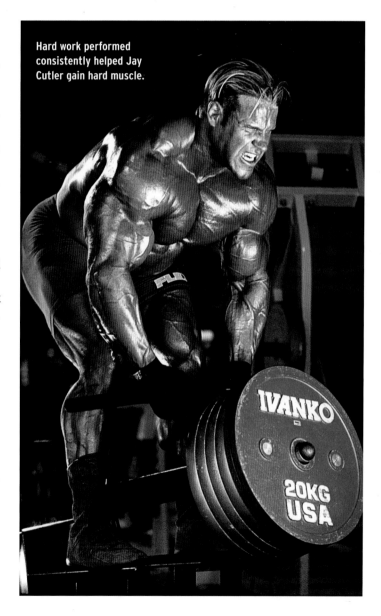

Hard work performed consistently helped Jay Cutler gain hard muscle.

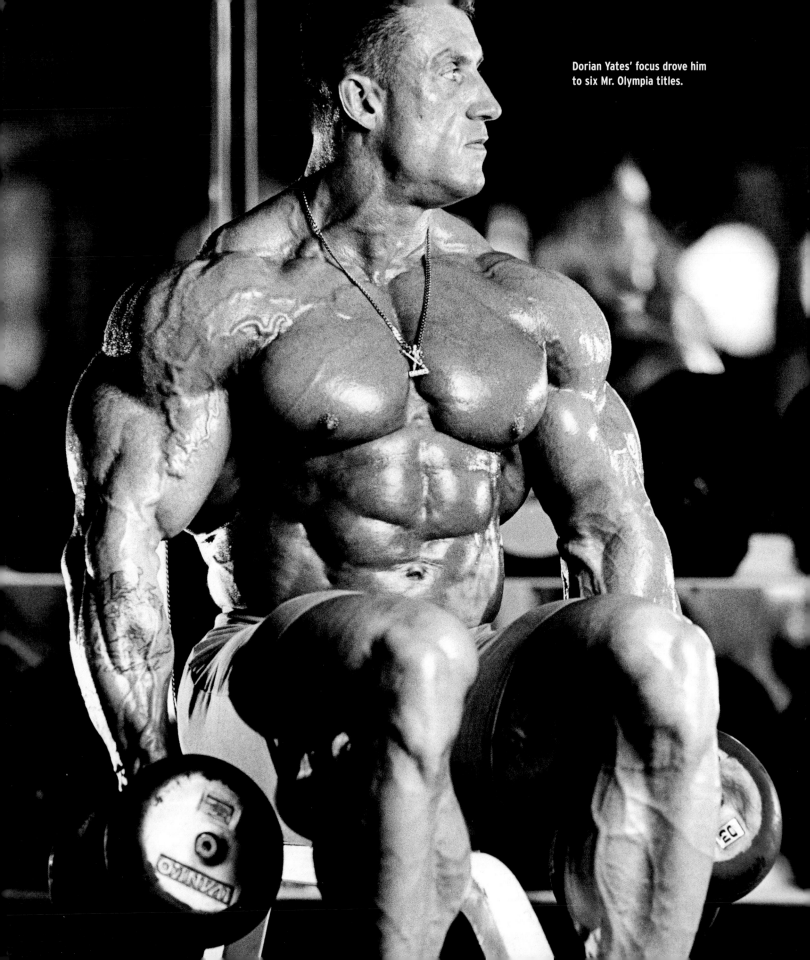

Dorian Yates' focus drove him to six Mr. Olympia titles.

Change Your Life for the BIGGER

Inspiration and focus are the keys to your bodybuilding success

Before you launch into the training programs contained here in this book and start throwing weights around with abandon, *FLEX* recommends that you do two things to start your program on the right track: First, settle back and read the entire book. This is a complex program, and it's our contention that you'll be able to make the most of it if you understand the full regimen from the outset. Reading the whole book will give you the big picture you need to make the most of your efforts. Of course, you'll need to revisit *HUGE* chapter by chapter as you go through the program — like we said, there's

a lot of info in this book, and you're going to want to get as much as you can from it.

Second, we want you to think about what you want to get from your personal bodybuilding program. Many people turn to bodybuilding for the individual challenge of simply getting bigger. By definition, bodybuilding represents a process of change and gradual improvement, but it's much more than simply the growth of your muscles. Bodybuilding is also a lifestyle that represents an environment in which you can directly control your own destiny in a positive sense. And that's what we'd like you to think about: What can bodybuilding do for you?

Without guidance, this may be a difficult question to answer before you even pick up a weight. Consider that, for many people, bodybuilding is the road to self-esteem; for others, it's a form of therapy used to turn their lives around after major

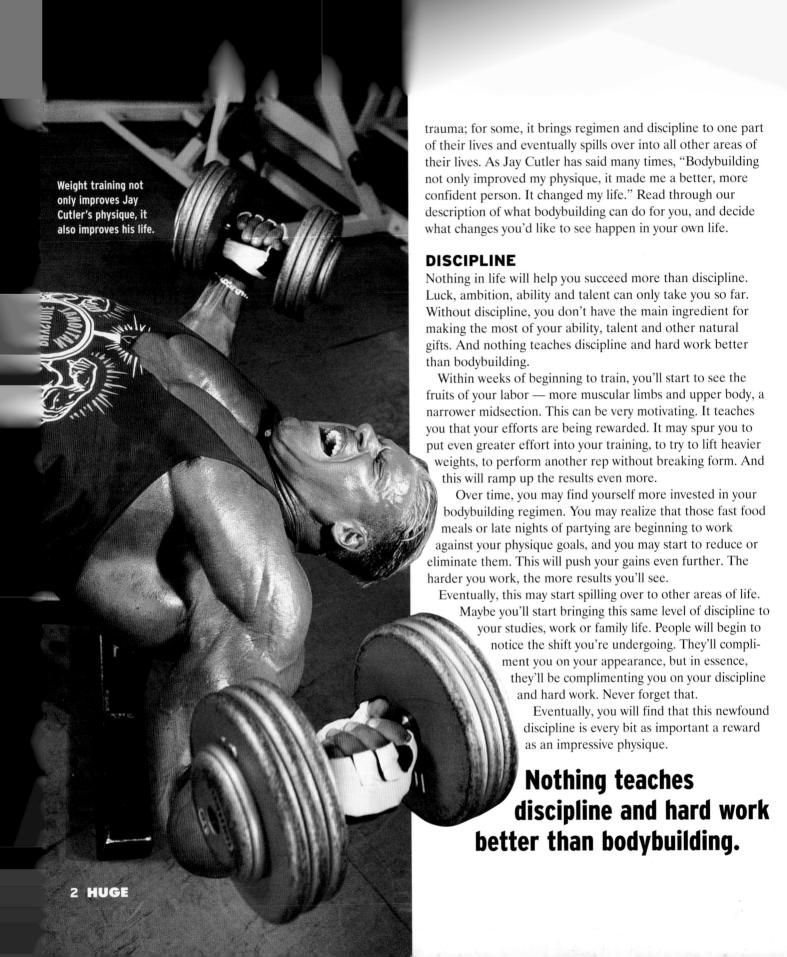

Weight training not only improves Jay Cutler's physique, it also improves his life.

trauma; for some, it brings regimen and discipline to one part of their lives and eventually spills over into all other areas of their lives. As Jay Cutler has said many times, "Bodybuilding not only improved my physique, it made me a better, more confident person. It changed my life." Read through our description of what bodybuilding can do for you, and decide what changes you'd like to see happen in your own life.

DISCIPLINE

Nothing in life will help you succeed more than discipline. Luck, ambition, ability and talent can only take you so far. Without discipline, you don't have the main ingredient for making the most of your ability, talent and other natural gifts. And nothing teaches discipline and hard work better than bodybuilding.

Within weeks of beginning to train, you'll start to see the fruits of your labor — more muscular limbs and upper body, a narrower midsection. This can be very motivating. It teaches you that your efforts are being rewarded. It may spur you to put even greater effort into your training, to try to lift heavier weights, to perform another rep without breaking form. And this will ramp up the results even more.

Over time, you may find yourself more invested in your bodybuilding regimen. You may realize that those fast food meals or late nights of partying are beginning to work against your physique goals, and you may start to reduce or eliminate them. This will push your gains even further. The harder you work, the more results you'll see.

Eventually, this may start spilling over to other areas of life. Maybe you'll start bringing this same level of discipline to your studies, work or family life. People will begin to notice the shift you're undergoing. They'll compliment you on your appearance, but in essence, they'll be complimenting you on your discipline and hard work. Never forget that.

Eventually, you will find that this newfound discipline is every bit as important a reward as an impressive physique.

Nothing teaches discipline and hard work better than bodybuilding.

CHANGE YOUR LIFE FOR THE BIGGER

Tenacity and discipline have helped King Kamali become a top pro bodybuilder.

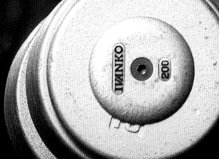
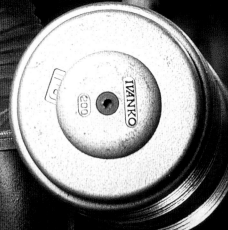

CHAPTER ONE

Günter Schlierkamp and Kevin Levrone have found bodybuilding success through intensity, motivation and discipline.

CHANGE YOUR LIFE FOR THE BIGGER

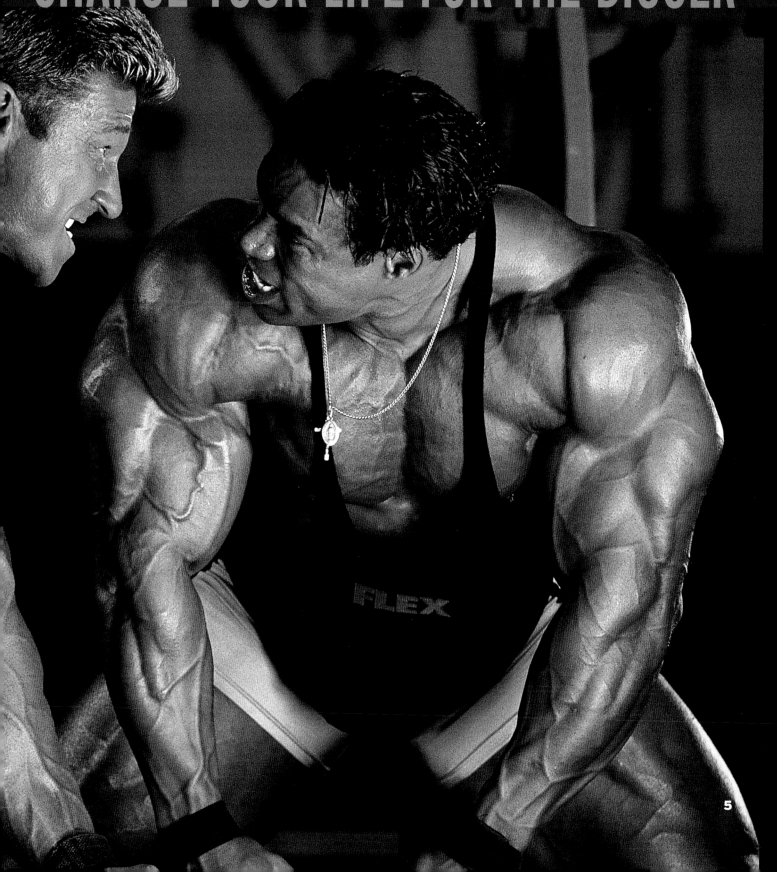

CHAPTER ONE

Bodybuilding is one of the cornerstones of Garrett Downing's life.

SELF-ESTEEM

Bodybuilding is a clear path to improving your attitude about yourself. When you apply the discipline and invest the time in yourself that bodybuilding requires, you are sending a subconscious message to yourself that you are important.

When you begin to eat healthy to support growth and recuperation, you are making a distinction between the quality foods you allow into your body and the unhealthy foods you have decided against. You are demonstrating a respect for your body that will manifest itself in a better appearance, but, more importantly, in feeling better and in being healthier.

As you make better choices with how you spend your time to accommodate your bodybuilding program, you'll find your attitude changing for the better. Many vices you might have indulged in previously will seem like a waste of time and effort, and you'll find yourself rejecting them. Over time, you'll notice a change in yourself and when you think back to the bad choices you used to make, you won't believe that was you! That comparison is evidence that you have gained self-esteem from your program.

IS BODYBUILDING A SPORT?

Like all sports, bodybuilding requires discipline and dedication. It requires training. But our answer to this question is, surprisingly, no. While bodybuilding has many of the elements of other sports, *FLEX* believes that bodybuilding is much more than just a game or contest. Football is a sport. Baseball is a sport. But compared to the millions of people who watch these sports, few actually participate in them.

Bodybuilding transcends being a sport because it is so highly participatory and because it is such an important part of bodybuilders' lives. While many fans of bodybuilding competitions are die-hard enthusiasts, the real love is in practicing it. Bodybuilding gives meaning to life by helping people lead more productive lives.

YOUR BIG BODYBUILDING PROGRAM

We hope this has provided some insight into what you can expect from bodybuilding and from this book itself. Identifying what you want to get from life — in addition to bigger muscles — will help you on your path to bodybuilding success. Whatever reason you have come to bodybuilding, one thing we can assure you of is that bodybuilding can be a force for positive change in your own life. *HUGE* will change your life. It will make you a bigger person in all senses.

Now, turn the page and get started.

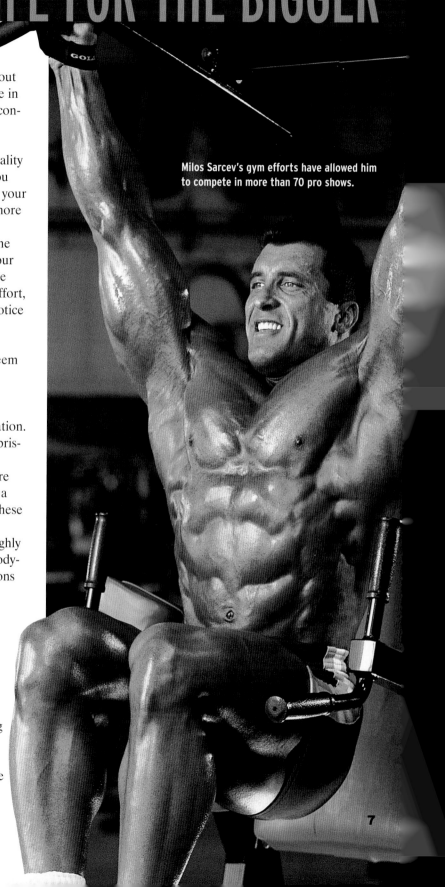

Milos Sarcev's gym efforts have allowed him to compete in more than 70 pro shows.

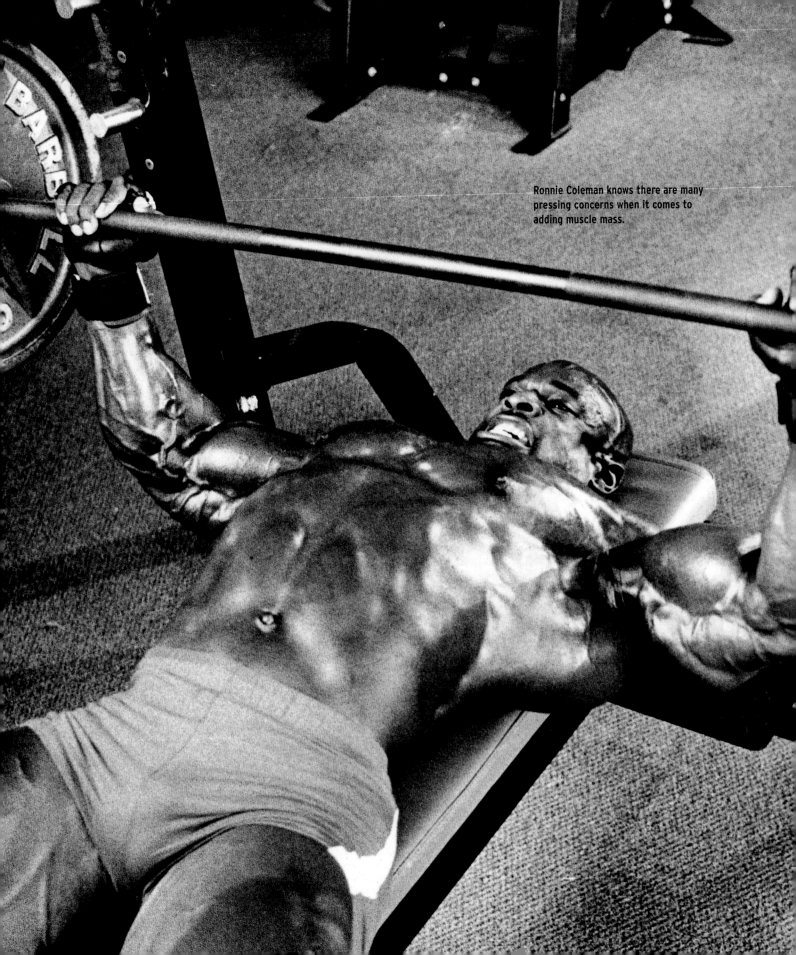

Ronnie Coleman knows there are many pressing concerns when it comes to adding muscle mass.

The First
FOUR WEEKS

A training program that will instill you with the basics of bodybuilding

Just as you cannot begin training for a marathon by actually running 26 miles, you can't start getting huge by working out like a top pro from day one. You first need to gradually introduce your muscles to the rigors and idiosyncrasies of lifting weights. So *FLEX* created this four-week introductory training program that will enable you and your physiology to become familiar with correct lifting technique — the "groove" of training — and breed safe habits that will ensure bodybuilding longevity.

This introductory program should be completed three times a week on nonconsecutive days (e.g., Monday, Wednesday, Friday) for four weeks. It's important to note that the first set of each exercise is a warm-up set, in which you lift 50% of the poundage you will use for the succeeding sets. For those remaining sets, you need to use a weight at which muscular failure would occur just beyond the 15-rep mark. Each exercise is to be performed with strict style. We deliberately stress that you do not work to failure (that comes in later programs) because the whole point of this beginning period is for you to develop good lifting style within your own strength capabilities. Do not do extra sets or exercises beyond the ones listed, or you may fall into the overtraining syndrome.

BASICS FIRST
The routine is made up of "basic" compound movements.

Basic exercises represent the best means of gaining mass quickly, and that's why they are the cornerstone of this program.

Basic exercises not only concentrate on working a major bodypart, but also call into play other surrounding muscle groups. For instance, the bench press (the basic exercise for chest) directly works the chest (pectoral) muscles while indirectly working the triceps and front-delt muscles.

The opposite of basic movements are isolation exercises. These exercises — by definition — isolate a specific muscle and do not involve the recruitment of secondary muscle groups. For example, an isolation exercise for front thighs (quads) is the leg extension. This movement works the quads and only the quads. In contrast, the basic movement for front thighs is the barbell squat, which uses the glutes, hamstrings and lower back as secondary muscle groups. Therefore, you can use heavier poundages while squatting, a basic movement, than you can while doing leg extensions, an isolation movement.

We include a basic movement for each of the four major bodyparts: quads, chest, back, shoulders. These are the powerhouse bodyparts, which can move the most weight and therefore trigger the optimum amount of muscle gain.

In short, basic exercises represent the best means of gaining mass quickly, and that's why they are the cornerstone of this program.

SAFE SETS

Follow the instructions for all exercises to the letter, and complete them in a controlled fashion. Don't jerk the weights, as this leads to injury. For further safety, wear a lifting belt to protect the injury-prone lower back. We advise you to wear the belt at all training times, apart from during abdominal and chest work. Loosen it between sets; have it tight only when actually working out.

We prescribe crunches and hyperextensions at the start of every workout. The lower back is probably the most injury-prone area for a bodybuilder. Although hyper-

INTRODUCTION PROGRAM

THE WARM-UP
Ten minutes on stationary bike or cardio alternative
Two to three minutes of stretching

WORKING SETS

BODYPART	EXERCISE	SETS	REPS
Abs	Forward crunches	3	15
Lower back	Hyperextensions	3	10
Thighs	Barbell squats	4	15
Chest	Barbell bench presses	4	15
Back	Barbell rows	4	15
Upper lats	Chins or lat pulldowns to the front	4	15
Shoulders	Seated military presses	4	15
Triceps	Close-grip bench presses	4	15
Biceps	Barbell curls	4	15

extensions directly strengthen the lower back, a strong and well-developed midsection also helps guard against lower-back problems because the abdominals work as stabilizer muscles in many basic exercises such as squats, rows and presses.

TRAINING TIPS

■ The priority is learning correct technique for each movement.

■ Do not train to failure: Use a poundage with which you can just complete the required number of reps.

■ Many beginners find it impossible to complete the required number of reps of chins, but get as many as you can. You will get stronger over time.

■ The first set of each exercise represents a warm-up. Lift 50% of the poundage you'll use on the remainder of your sets. (This does not apply to nonweighted crunches, hyperextensions and chins. For these exercises, do the required number of reps.)

■ Rest a couple of minutes after each set so that you attempt each in fresh condition.

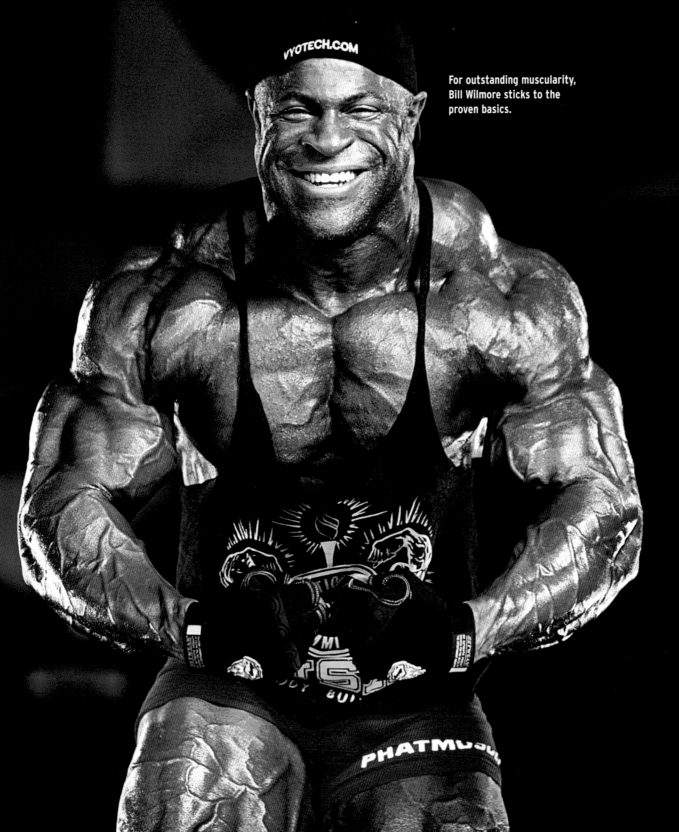

For outstanding muscularity, Bill Wilmore sticks to the proven basics.

If you want the quickest route to
ab development, Lee Priest says
crunches are essential.

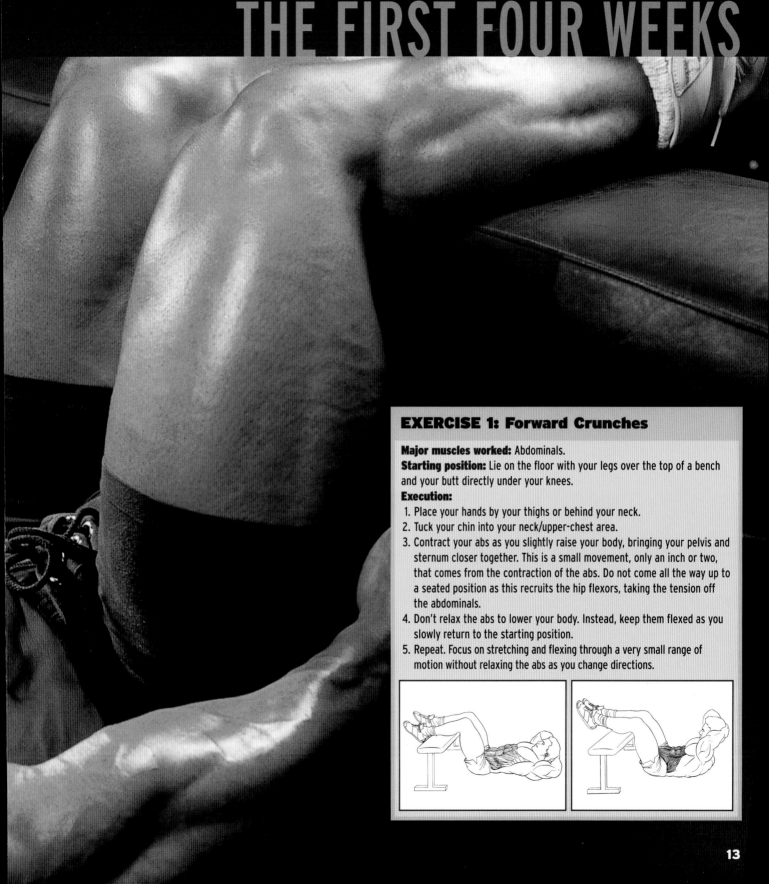

EXERCISE 1: Forward Crunches

Major muscles worked: Abdominals.

Starting position: Lie on the floor with your legs over the top of a bench and your butt directly under your knees.

Execution:

1. Place your hands by your thighs or behind your neck.
2. Tuck your chin into your neck/upper-chest area.
3. Contract your abs as you slightly raise your body, bringing your pelvis and sternum closer together. This is a small movement, only an inch or two, that comes from the contraction of the abs. Do not come all the way up to a seated position as this recruits the hip flexors, taking the tension off the abdominals.
4. Don't relax the abs to lower your body. Instead, keep them flexed as you slowly return to the starting position.
5. Repeat. Focus on stretching and flexing through a very small range of motion without relaxing the abs as you change directions.

Core strength is at the core
of Milos Sarcev's training.

EXERCISE 2: Hyperextensions

Major muscles worked: Spinal erectors, hamstrings and gluteals.

Starting position: Mount the bench facing downward with the pad at the top of your pelvis. Keep tension in your lower back throughout the movement, while you keep your head in a neutral position and your arms across your chest. Your knees should be slightly bent and your leg muscles locked. This exercise is performed in three phases: the first focusing on spinal erectors, the second focusing on hamstrings, and the third focusing on using spinal erectors, hamstrings and gluteals in sync. It's important to think about the target muscles as you work through each phase.

Execution:

1. Round your upper back slightly and rotate your trunk downward about two inches, feeling the stretch in your spinal erectors while maintaining a slight arch in your lower back.
2. Raise your upper body – past the starting position if possible – by flexing your spinal erectors (arching your back) and abs. Repeat 10 times. This is the first phase of the exercise.
3. Bend your trunk downward, lowering it about five inches while maintaining the tension in your lower back and hamstrings. Do not go so low that you relax the muscles of your lower back.
4. Pause at the bottom of the motion on every rep to avoid using momentum to raise your body.
5. Flex your back and pull from the back of your ankles, feeling the hamstrings working. Repeat 10 times to complete the second phase.
6. Begin the final phase of the exercise. Use a full range of motion: i.e., from straight body to a jackknife (45-degree) angle. Complete the movement slowly, continuing to feel the flexion in your lower back and hams. Add a gluteal contraction as you drive your hips into the bench and return to the upright position. Perform 10 reps.

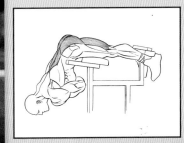
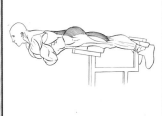

Sarcev performs squats because they are the single best exercise for stimulating muscle growth.

EXERCISE 3: Barbell Squats

Major muscles worked: Quadriceps, hamstrings, hips and glutes.
Secondary muscles: Calves.
Starting position: Step under the bar. Shoulders are down and back, so that the bar rests on the muscles of your upper back. Make sure the bar is not touching a bone in the spine. Use a comfortable hand grip; generally speaking, the wider the grip, the more stable the movement. Chest is up and out. Fix your gaze on an object at eye level, and keep it there throughout the movement. This ensures that your head will remain in proper position.
Execution:

1. Place your feet slightly wider than shoulder width, though this will vary slightly depending on flexibility and comfort; for instance, if it's hard to squat flat-footed, space your feet a little farther apart – this keeps the lower back tight.
2. Arch your lower back. Keep your heels flat on the floor and think about pushing down through your heels throughout the movement.
3. Take a deep breath and release it as you begin the ascent.
4. As you begin to descend, consciously think of "sitting back into the squat" rather than just thrusting your knees forward to activate the descent. Keep your hips locked and lower back arched.
5. Slowly descend and squat as deep as possible – until there's no longer a sensation of stretching the hamstrings – while staying in control of the weight. Knees should never extend past the toes. Again, think of "sitting back into the squat."
6. At the midpoint, drive down with your heels, squeeze your glutes and push up, pulling your hips forward on the return to the starting position.

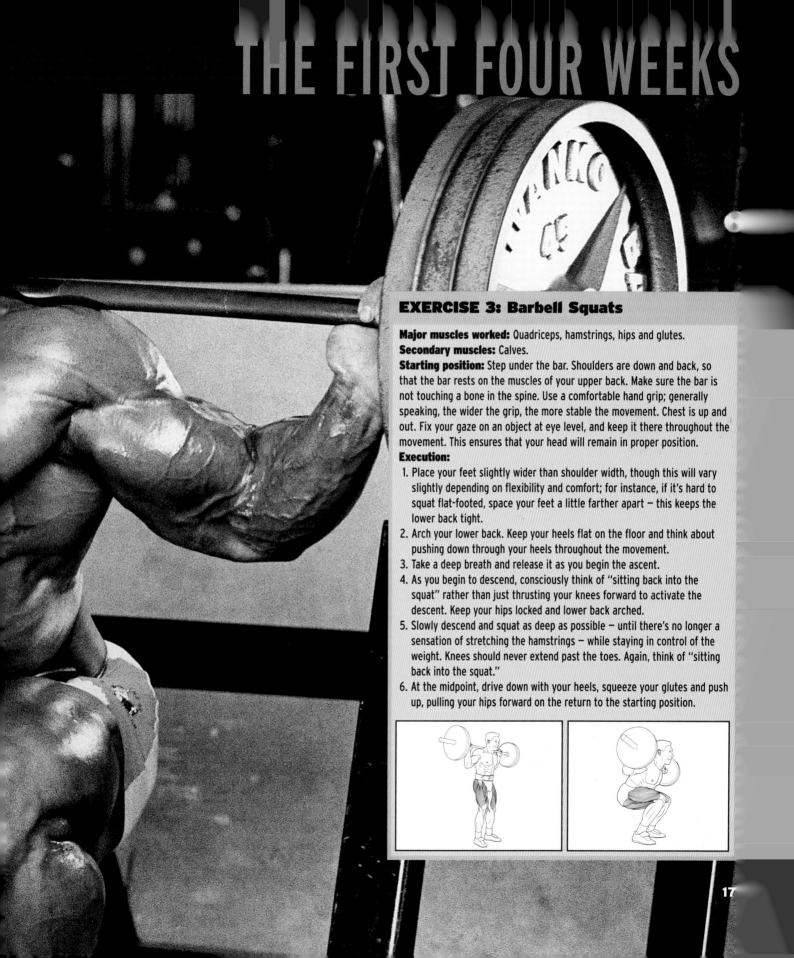

CHAPTER TWO

Kevin Levrone has relied on bench presses to build impressive pectorals.

EXERCISE 4: Barbell Bench Presses

Major muscles worked: The entire chest group.

Secondary muscles: Deltoids and triceps.

Starting position: Lie on a bench, feet on the floor, toes out. Grasp a barbell with a grip 12 inches wider than shoulder width. Thumbs should be over the bar, chest should be up and out, shoulders down and back.

Execution:

1. Before starting to lower the bar, take a deep breath, hold it as the bar descends, then exhale as you start the ascent.
2. Slowly lower the bar to just below nipple level, focusing on feeling a stretch in your pecs. Don't think about the weight itself; instead, concentrate on flexing the muscle. Don't arch your back.
3. Let the bar just touch your chest – don't bounce it – and then, keeping the pecs tensed and with no assistance from body movement, slowly drive the bar back up to just short of lockout. Adopting the nonlockout style keeps the tension directly on your pecs and doesn't allow your triceps to take over the major pressure of the weight.
4. From the nonlockout position, repeat the movement.

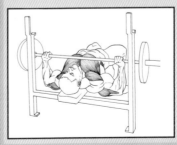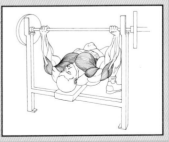

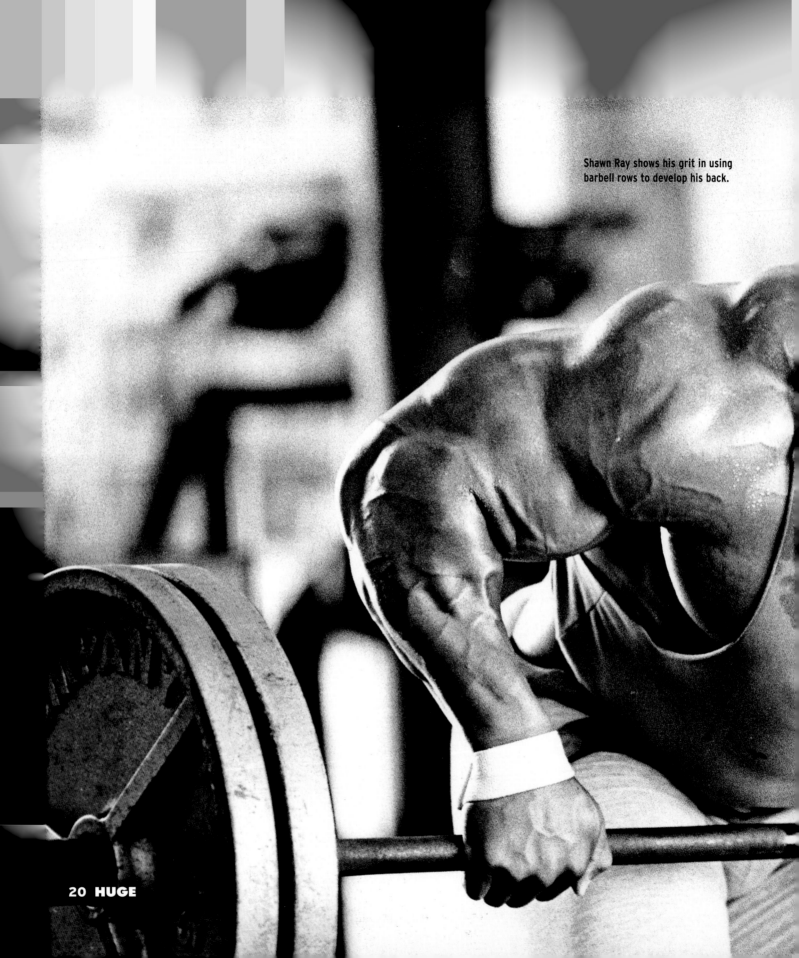

Shawn Ray shows his grit in using barbell rows to develop his back.

EXERCISE 5: Barbell Rows

Major muscles worked: Lats, rhomboids and teres major.

Secondary muscles: Rear delts and traps.

Starting position: With the barbell on the floor, bend and grasp the bar with a thumbs-over-the-bar overhand grip. Use wrist wraps, if necessary, to assist with the grip. With your knees slightly bent, bend your upper body forward. Your shoulders should be thrust back, your upper and lower back arched and locked.

Execution:

1. With only your arms moving, concentrate on pulling with your lats as you drive your elbows back.
2. Keeping your elbows close to your sides, pull the bar to ab or lower-chest level and squeeze your lats as you reach the midpoint.
3. Lower to the starting position, and let your arms hang fully extended as you feel a stretch in your middle back.

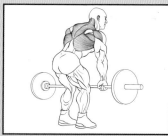 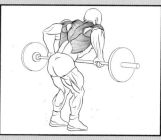

CHAPTER TWO

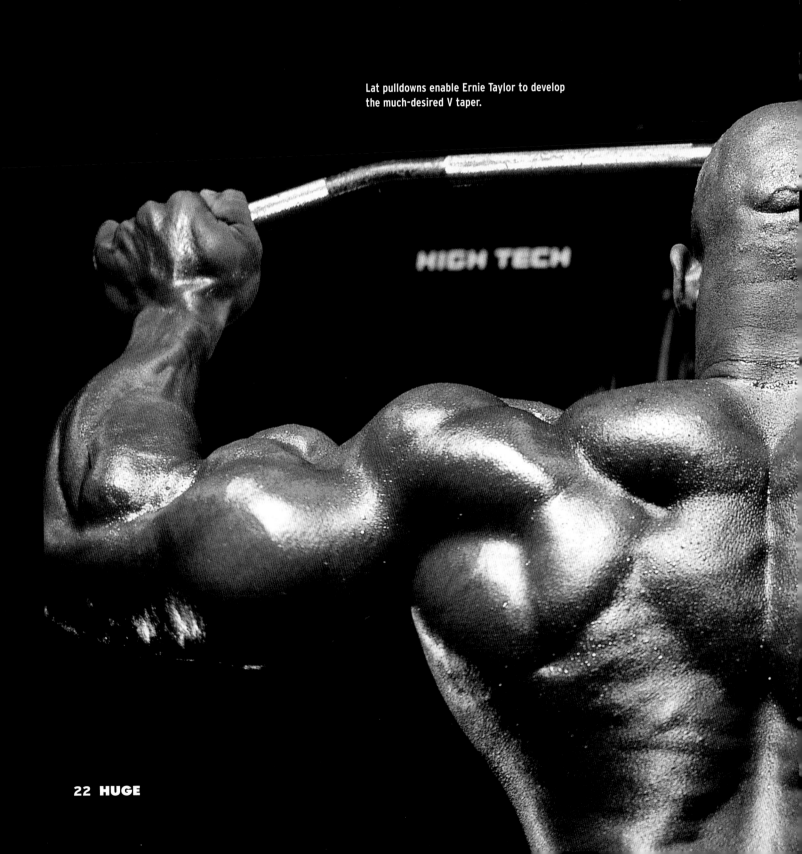

Lat pulldowns enable Ernie Taylor to develop the much-desired V taper.

HIGH TECH

EXERCISE 6: Lat Pulldowns to the Front

(as a substitute for chins, if necessary)

Major muscles worked: Lats and teres major.

Secondary muscles: Rear delts, rhomboids, teres major, triceps and pecs.

Starting position: Sit in the lat machine and take an overhand grip about 12 inches beyond shoulder width. With your arms fully extended, puff up your chest, arch your back and lean slightly backward.

Execution:

1. Using just the power of your lats, and with only your arms moving, begin to pull the bar down toward your upper chest.
2. Pull your elbows as far down and back as possible, until the bar touches your chest.
3. Hold at that midpoint position, and squeeze your lats for one second before slowly returning to the starting position.

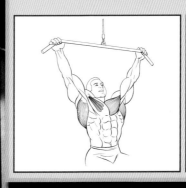
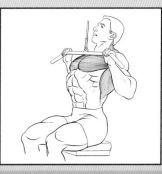

EXERCISE 7: Chins

Major muscles worked: Lats.

Secondary muscles: Rear delts, rhomboids, teres major, biceps and pecs.

Starting position: Grasp an overhead bar with a wider than shoulder-width thumbs-over-the-bar overhand grip. Use wrist straps, if necessary, to assist with the grip and minimize biceps involvement in the movement. Hang from the bar, and cross your feet to stabilize your hips and protect your spine.

Execution:

1. From the fully extended hanging position, pull with the power of your lats and drive your elbows as far back as possible to raise your body. Bring your head above bar level and your upper chest to bar level.

2. Hang in that position for a moment, and squeeze with your lats and midback muscles.

3. Slowly lower to the starting position, feeling your lats stretch as you descend.

Sarcev knows that chins are the ultimate weight-resistance exercise.

Darrem Charles uses military presses to stimulate all three deltoid heads.

EXERCISE 8: Seated Military Presses

Major muscles worked: Front and lateral deltoids.
Secondary muscles: Rear deltoids and traps.
Starting position: Assuming a slightly-wider-than-shoulder-width thumbs-over-the-bar grip, place the barbell along the line of your clavicles.

Execution:
1. Keep your lower back tight, upper back arched and chest out.
2. At the start position, keep your elbows in close to your sides with your shoulders back. With your upper body remaining stable, start to push the bar up, moving your elbows out to your sides as the bar is raised. Feel and control your deltoid muscles.
3. Press the bar almost to arms' length overhead. Don't lock out at the top; this keeps the pressure on the deltoid muscles.
4. Slowly lower the weight to the starting position, keeping the stress on your delts at all times.

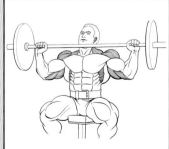
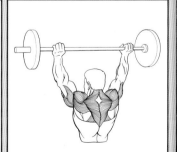

EXERCISE 9: Close-Grip Bench Presses

Major muscles worked: Triceps.
Secondary muscles worked: Pecs and front delts.
Starting position: Lie flat on a bench and grasp an overhead bar with a grip slightly less than shoulder width.
Execution:

1. Hold the bar overhead and, keeping your elbows at your sides, begin to slowly lower the weight.
2. Keeping your elbows tucked in, bring the bar down until it touches your lower chest.
3. Keeping your elbows in, and without bouncing the weight, push the bar back up to the starting position.

With a straight or cambered bar, close-grip bench presses have been an integral part in Levrone's triceps development.

EXERCISE 10: Barbell Curls

Major muscles worked: Biceps.

Secondary muscles: Front delts, forearms and lower back.

Starting position: Assume a shoulder-width curl grip and stand with your arms fully extended and the barbell resting against your thighs.

Execution:

1. With only your lower arms moving (there should be no movement of your upper arms or the rest of your body), curl the weight upward until your knuckles almost make contact with your front delts.
2. At this point, pause and squeeze your biceps for a count of one.
3. Slowly return to the starting position.

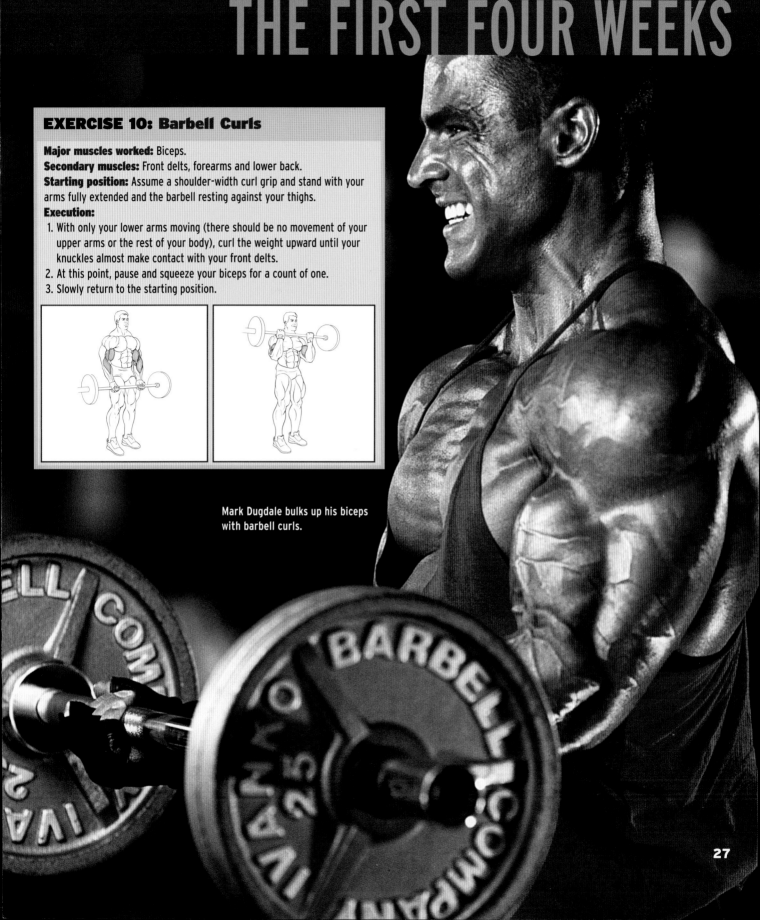

Mark Dugdale bulks up his biceps with barbell curls.

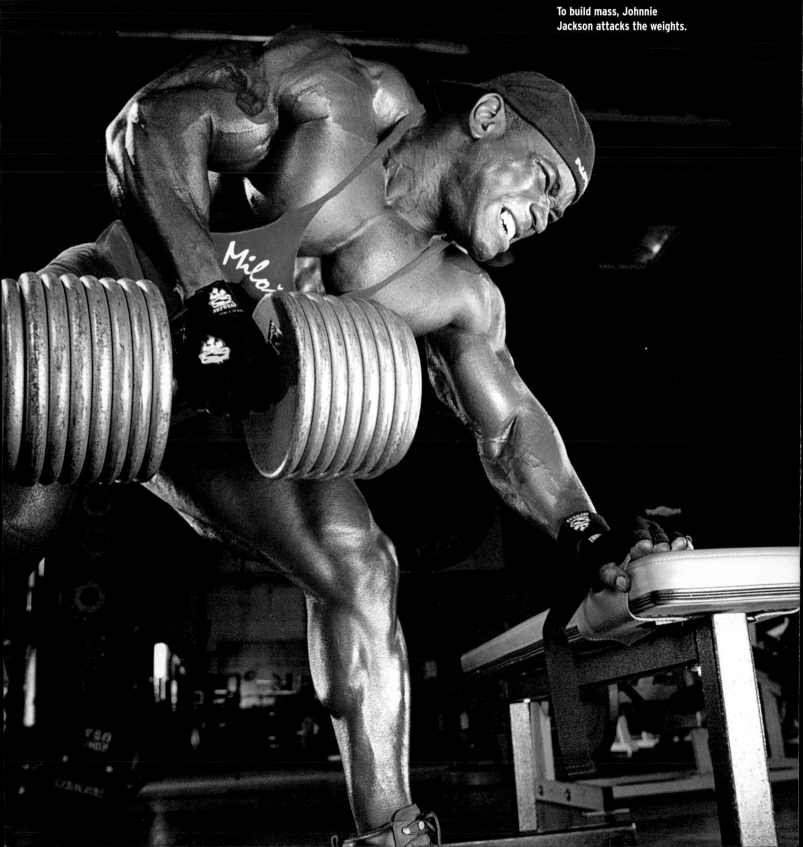

To build mass, Johnnie Jackson attacks the weights.

Mass ATTACK

Explore the full potential of your inner bodybuilder with our muscle-building program

It's your year to become Mr. Huge.

How do we know this? Because we have the technology. We have the science. We have decades of experience, and we've put it all together in the ultimate comprehensive bodybuilding program. Beginning with this chapter and continuing through the end of the book, our program constitutes a step-by-step guide on how to build and retain quality muscle.

FUTURE SHOCK: YOU WILL GROW!

The program begins by demanding two elements that may sound contradictory: a thinking man's approach to training and nutrition, combined with brutal animalistic intensity. That's actually the FLEX credo in a nutshell, but this program puts it all together.

HUGE is a yearlong journey that you'll begin immediately. It's accompanied by cutting-edge nutrition guidelines and other tricks of the trade to push you further along your evolutionary trail. Here's a brief rundown of the program's key elements.

BEGINNING: THE PHASES

In this chapter, we'll outline the first three-month chunk of the program. It consists of two phases, each lasting six weeks, with a week of rest in between.

PHASE ONE: The first six weeks retrains your neuromuscular system to learn the correct stimulus response to resistance training. It consists of high sets and reps, using moderate weight (see the exercise charts that accompany this article). At the beginning, it's important that you rest two minutes between sets. You will gradually decrease the rest time and increase the amount of weight you lift as you progress.

Phase one teaches you to master perfect form and build your conditioning base. These first six weeks are crucial for rewiring your neuromuscular system and creating a synergistic mind-body functioning that primes you for increased weights and intensity for the next six-week phase.

PHASE TWO: After phase one, rest one week to reset your system and prepare it for phase two. This six-week period instructs you to increase weight, reduce reps and deal with the pain zone. The exercises and training split remain the same, however, for both phases.

THE SPLIT

In phases one and two, you will forgo aerobics and concentrate solely on weight training. This is a two-on/one-off/

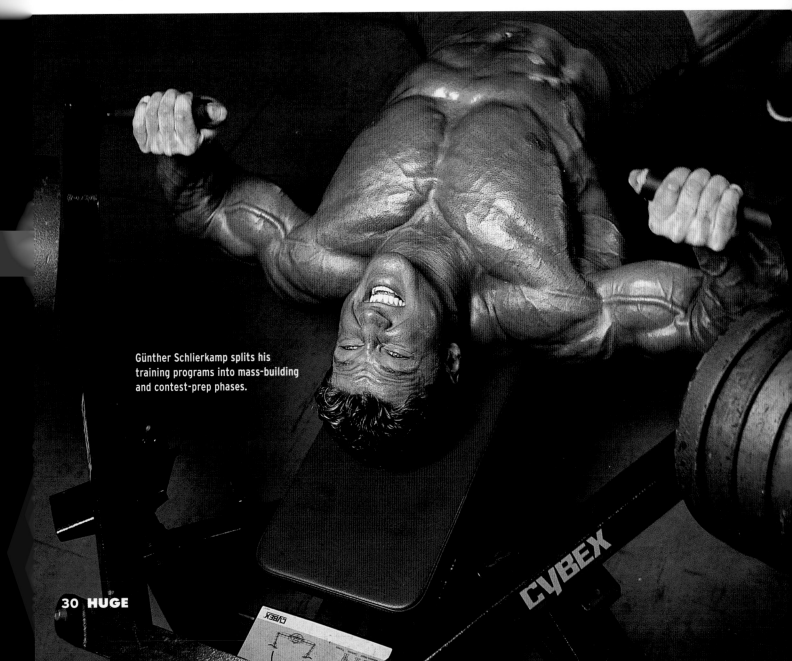

Günther Schlierkamp splits his training programs into mass-building and contest-prep phases.

two-on/two-off weekly split. Here's an example of this split pattern.

Monday: abs and legs
Tuesday: back and arms
Wednesday: rest
Thursday: chest and delts
Friday: abs and legs
Saturday and Sunday: rest

Following this protocol, you'll train the entire body four times every three weeks. Though abdominal training is called for, you'll go light on abs for now, merely strengthening your midsection for its role as a main stabilizer during most power movements as you increase weight and intensity while moving through the program.

Don't get clever by switching things up right away. There's plenty of time for personalizing the program in future months. For now, you need to follow our system to the letter to ensure that you're laying the necessary foundation.

There can be no weak points if you're going to build an overall awesome physique, because muscle builds systemically, not in spots. You can target improvements, but mass gains are subject to an overall neuromuscular response and the whims of your genetics. The key is to get the most out of your genetics with the tools available. That's what the programs in this book are designed to do.

THE EXERCISES

Starting on page 36, we illustrate and explain the proper form for executing all the exercises. These exercises are set in stone—for now, anyway. We didn't come up with this collection of movements off the tops of our heads. We're sure these are the exercises that, when used in concert, will provide your body with what it requires to stimulate its best long-term gains.

Not surprisingly, you'll be asked to do compound free-weight movements, bread-and-butter type exercises that you may dread doing. Don't worry if you've never felt comfortable doing deadlifts and squats, for instance. We'll teach you how to do them safely and correctly, and since we begin with moderate weight, you will not rush into achieving personal bests with movements that you may not be comfortable doing. The idea is to train your neuromuscular pathways and your psyche, so that these foundation exercises will be hardwired into your entire physiological system. Your first goal in this program is to master form and feel. Heavy lifting will follow.

THE CYCLE

Young bodybuilders often make the mistake of overtraining when they try to put on size. To achieve success on the program you should limit your training to four days a week.

The schedule in the exercise chart shows you how to set up your workouts to get the best results for every bodypart. On this timetable, you'll train each bodypart four times in three weeks. The three workouts rotate so that you tackle a different one after two days of rest at the beginning of each week. (See the "Workout Rotation" chart on page 47.) This allows for maximal recovery, enabling you to intensify the subsequent workout.

At the end of week three, start the rotation over. Complete the cycle twice for phase one of the program, a total of six weeks. After a week of rest, you'll begin phase two, which will also consist of two three-week rotations. The sets and reps will change for most of the exercises in the second phase.

FAILURE–*NOT!*

The program may throw you at first by specifying not going to failure on your sets—at least, failure as you know it. Misdirected stress and too many injuries result from using bad form. You hear it over and over from FLEX, but it's still the most abused aspect of training. As every experienced bodybuilder and training expert worth his biceps will tell you, make perfect form a priority because it's so important.

In the chapters that follow, we'll introduce intensity and shock techniques, but concentrate on achieving perfect reps for now. For your sets, use a poundage with which you will just manage to eke out your target reps before hitting failure. For example, if your target is 15 reps, you should reach that quota with perfect form but be unable to do a 16th rep with perfect form.

THE DISCIPLINE TO REST

As you'll notice in the training split, you'll take weekends off. It's important for you to stick to this split, to take these days to recharge, to keep your head from becoming too focused on the gym. There's nothing more pathetic than being one of those guys who hangs out at the gym during his rest days. The weekend (or whatever days your two-off lands on) is your time.

That doesn't mean you screw up everything you've done over the week by becoming Caligula and overindulging in sloth and sweets. Instead, play hoops, ski or participate in some other athletic activity you enjoy.

Also, get plenty of sleep. Although, with this program, you spend a lot of time in the gym at first (due to the two-minute rest between sets), you eventually will reduce your workout time as you increase weight and intensity. It's important, however, for you to allow your body to heal from the beautiful damage you've done to it while training. Sleep, in particular, is a time when goodies such as growth hormones are released in your body. Take advantage by getting enough rest. That's when you grow.

EAT IT UP!

When you get right down to it, nutrition is as important as training. Chapter 6 includes the intricacies of protein cycling, along with definitive meal plans. This no-bull effective eating strategy will enable you to get the correct amounts of nutrients in your system at the optimum moments. In upcoming chapters, we'll provide more specific supplementing guidelines for phases such as cutting, but get the basic mass-building nutrition foundation established first. Everything builds from there.

TIME TO GET HARDCORE

We assume if you're holding this book, you're ready to join the hardcore. If you want to get big and cut, and learn how to stay that way by mastering the tools to do so, this program is for you. If you think this system won't work, we challenge you to try the program for a few months, following it as prescribed. Then just try to tell us it's inadequate! We guarantee you'll love it so much, you'll stick with it.

You've got to trust us. We're taking over your training and nutrition for now. Later, you'll get more leeway, but for the time being, we're boss. Follow the plan.

It's not as if you're climbing Mount Everest, and it's not brain surgery. It takes dedication—and the harder you work, the more you'll get out of it—but this program is not designed to break you in half. It's a steady, progressive and effective program. No shortcuts. No magic pills. Consistent gains are the best way to become an accomplished bodybuilder. Too many guys try it the wrong way, the easy way, and they burn out in a couple of years. We've seen it happen many times.

Use this book, build your foundation, and start growing now.

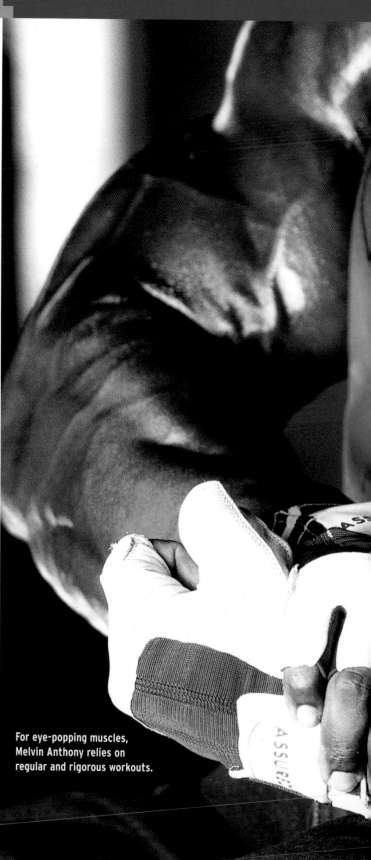

For eye-popping muscles, Melvin Anthony relies on regular and rigorous workouts.

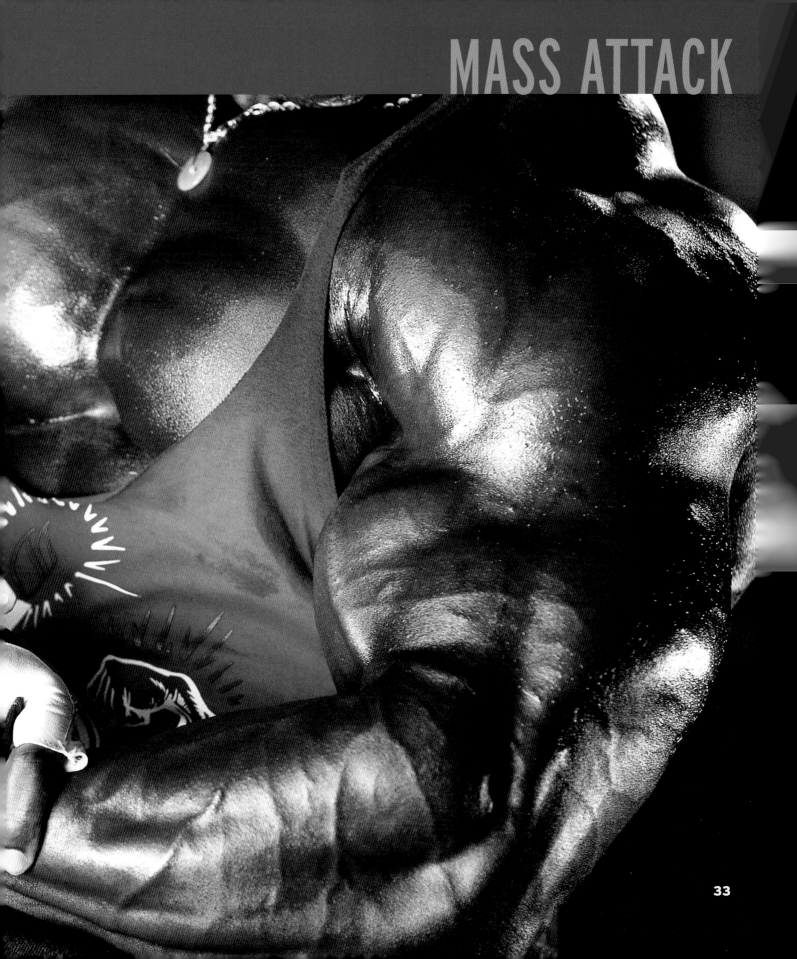

Anthony uses pre-planned rep schemes to add muscle mass.

THE FIRST THREE MONTHS

EXERCISE	PHASE ONE SETS X REPS	PHASE TWO SETS X REPS
WORKOUT ONE		
ABDOMINALS		
Lying leg raises	2 x 20	2 x 20
Forward crunches*	2 x 20	2 x 20
CALVES		
Standing calf raises	5 x 15	5 x 8-10
HAMSTRINGS		
Lying leg curls	5 x 12	5 x 8
QUADRICEPS		
Leg extensions	5 x 15	4 x 8
Barbell squats*	5 x 15	3 x 6-8
Leg presses	5 x 15	3 x 10
WORKOUT TWO		
CHEST		
Bench presses*	5 x 12	4 x 6
Incline dumbbell presses	5 x 12	3 x 8
Flat-bench flyes	5 x 12	3 x 8
SHOULDERS		
Seated front military presses*	5 x 10	5 x 5
Rear laterals on an incline bench	5 x 12	3 x 8
Seated dumbbell side laterals	5 x 12	3 x 8
TRAPEZIUS		
Dumbbell shrugs	5 x 10	4 x 6
WORKOUT THREE		
BACK		
Deadlifts	5 x 8	5 x 4-6
Bent rows*	5 x 12	3 x 8
Close-grip pulldowns to the front	5 x 12	3 x 8
TRICEPS		
Close-grip bench presses*	5 x 12	5 x 8
Triceps pushdowns	5 x 12	5 x 8
BICEPS		
Barbell curls*	5 x 12	5 x 6
Incline dumbbell curls	5 x 12	5 x 6

NOTES

For every bodypart (abs excepted), warm up by performing a light set of 25 reps of the first exercise. Use proper form. Do not train to failure: Use poundages with which you will be just able to reach your rep target before hitting failure.

*For descriptions of these exercises, see Chapter 2 "The First Four Weeks."

TIME MACHINE

This program has been carefully constructed to give you ultimate gains over the course of a year. The exercise selection, training frequency, and set-and-rep schemes have been specifically selected to allow for maximal recovery. One other aspect you must address in your training is the amount of rest you take between sets.

The amount of rest you provide your body is an often overlooked component of training. Bodybuilders frequently take as much rest as they need in order to lift as much weight as possible during the next set. This program asks you to challenge your muscles by progressively shortening your rest to place increasing demands on your muscles to allow maximal results.

In the first week, rest two minutes between each set as your body adjusts to higher reps during this new program. Each subsequent week, reduce your rest between sets by 10 seconds. For instance, the second week, rest for 110 seconds; the third week, rest for 100 seconds. Continue reducing your rest period until you are resting only about 70 seconds between sets for the sixth week.

The amount of rest you provide your body is an often overlooked component of training.

Reduced rest time is a more important element of this program than increased weight, because it trains your muscle fibers to endure the increased demands placed on them. While your aim is also to increase weight while maintaining the set-and-rep scheme, make certain you prioritize adhering to the time constraints of your rest period.

One of the obvious benefits of reducing your rest time is that your workouts will get progressively shorter as you advance through the program. You'll be doing more work in less time. That's what the pros call intensity.

WORKOUT ROTATION

WEEK	Monday	Tuesday	Thursday	Friday
One	One	Two	Three	One
Two	Two	Three	One	Two
Three	Three	One	Two	Three

Note: Rest on Sunday, Wednesday and Saturday

The Exercises

To isolate the lower abs, Tevita Aholelei employs lying leg raises.

Lying Leg Raises

Target area: Lower abdominals

Technique:

1. Lie on a bench with your glutes flat against the bench and your legs straight out in front of you.
2. Keeping your upper torso flat and legs straight, slowly raise your legs until they're at a 45-degree angle to the bench.
3. Pause for a second, then slowly return to the starting position.

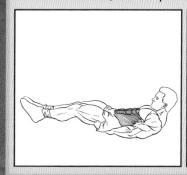 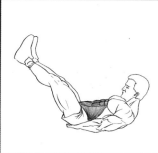

Standing Calf Raises

Target area: Total calf area

Technique:

1. Stand on a calf-raise machine with only your toes on the block.
2. Bend your knees slightly, with your torso and legs in a fixed position, then slowly lower your heels as far as comfortably possible.
3. Raise your heels—keeping your body straight—and push upward until you are standing on your tiptoes.
4. Hold for the contraction and return to the starting position.

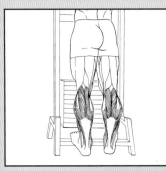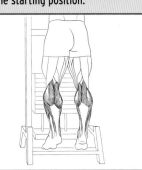

Mike Matarazzo raised the bar on calves development.

Jay Cutler knows that all leg muscles deserve individual attention.

Lying Leg Curls

Target area: Hamstrings (leg biceps)

Technique:

1. Lie facedown on the bench of a leg-curl machine and hook your heels under the footpads.
2. Making sure that your hips are flush against the bench, raise your heels until you can no longer pull any farther forward.
3. Lower the weight, slowly and under control, to return to the starting position.

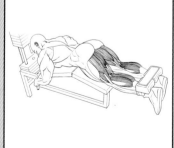 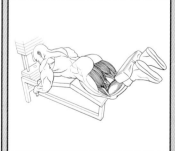

Leg Extensions

Target area: Quadriceps

Technique:

1. Sit on a leg-extension machine and place the tops of your feet under the footpads.
2. Keep your lower back supported against the seatback. Using only the power of your quadriceps, slowly lift your lower legs until the knee joints reach the lockout position.
3. Pause for the contraction, then slowly return to the starting position. Never rely on momentum to lift the weight or you will risk injury to your knee joints.

Note: This is an ideal way to warm up the quads for the heavy squats and leg presses to follow.

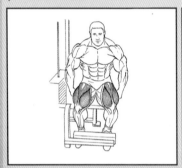
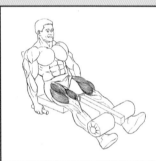

Leg extensions are a favorite thigh fry for Claude Groulx.

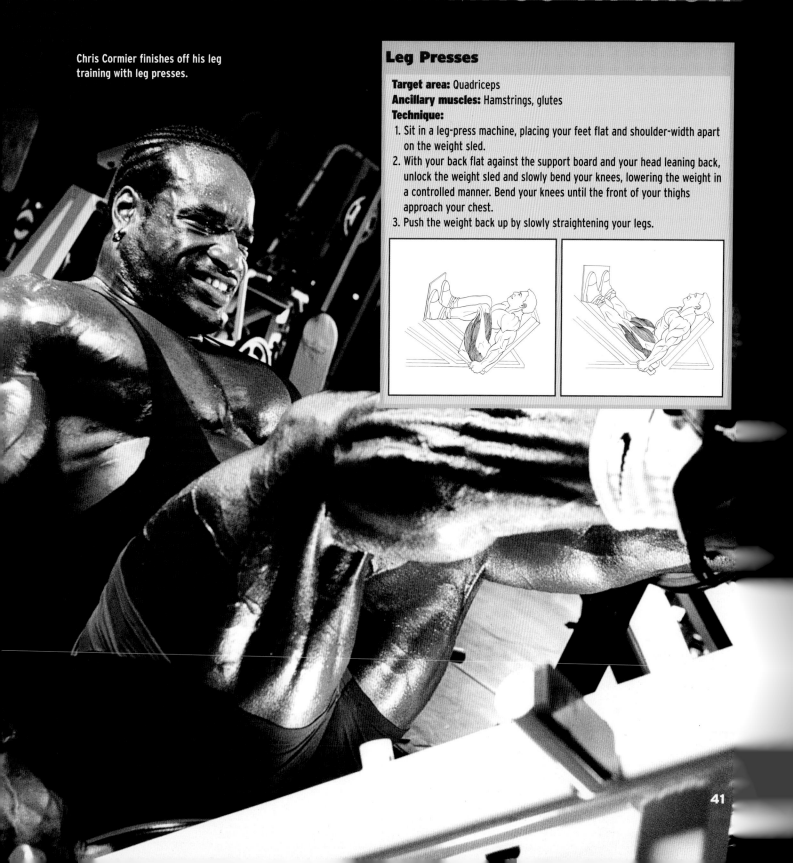

Chris Cormier finishes off his leg training with leg presses.

Leg Presses

Target area: Quadriceps

Ancillary muscles: Hamstrings, glutes

Technique:

1. Sit in a leg-press machine, placing your feet flat and shoulder-width apart on the weight sled.
2. With your back flat against the support board and your head leaning back, unlock the weight sled and slowly bend your knees, lowering the weight in a controlled manner. Bend your knees until the front of your thighs approach your chest.
3. Push the weight back up by slowly straightening your legs.

Incline Dumbbell Presses

Target area: Upper and outer pectorals
Ancillary muscles: Lower and middle pectorals, triceps, front delts
Technique:

1. Lie on an adjustable bench with the back support set at a 45-degree incline.
2. Grasp a pair of dumbbells and hold them at arm's length overhead—keep your thumb knuckles facing each other throughout the movement.
3. With elbows pointing outward, slowly lower the dumbbells until your hands are past pec level. The extended range of motion that dumbbells promote allows for greater stress on the outer pecs.
4. From this bottom position, press the dumbbells back up to the top.

e dumbbell presses are a
exercise in Kevin Levrone's
development. Dennis
s lends a hand.

Flat-Bench Flyes

Target area: The overall pectorals, with emphasis on the outer pecs
Ancillary muscles: Biceps, front delts
Technique:

1. Lie on a flat bench with the dumbbells held overhead at arm's length, palms facing each other.
2. Bend your arms slightly to reduce the pressure on the elbow joints. Maintain this bent-elbow position throughout the exercise.
3. Following a wide arc, lower the dumbbells out to the sides and down to chest level or below.
4. Relying on the power of your pecs, return the weights to the starting position.
5. The flye movement is often compared to hugging a tree—use this concept to help you stay clean and precise with the execution of the lift.

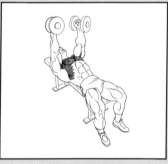
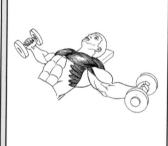

Ronnie Coleman incorporates flyes into his training because they are the best isolation move for developing pecs.

Rear Laterals on an Incline Bench

Target area: Rear delts

Technique:

1. Lie facedown on an incline bench set at a 45-degree angle and grasp a dumbbell in each hand.
2. Raise the dumbbells outward in an arc (vertically from the floor); do not turn or tilt the dumbbells.
3. Raise the dumbbells to a point where the backs of your hands are just above the level of the uppermost part of your delts.
4. Hold for a second before slowly lowering the weights to the starting position.

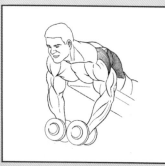
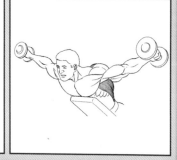

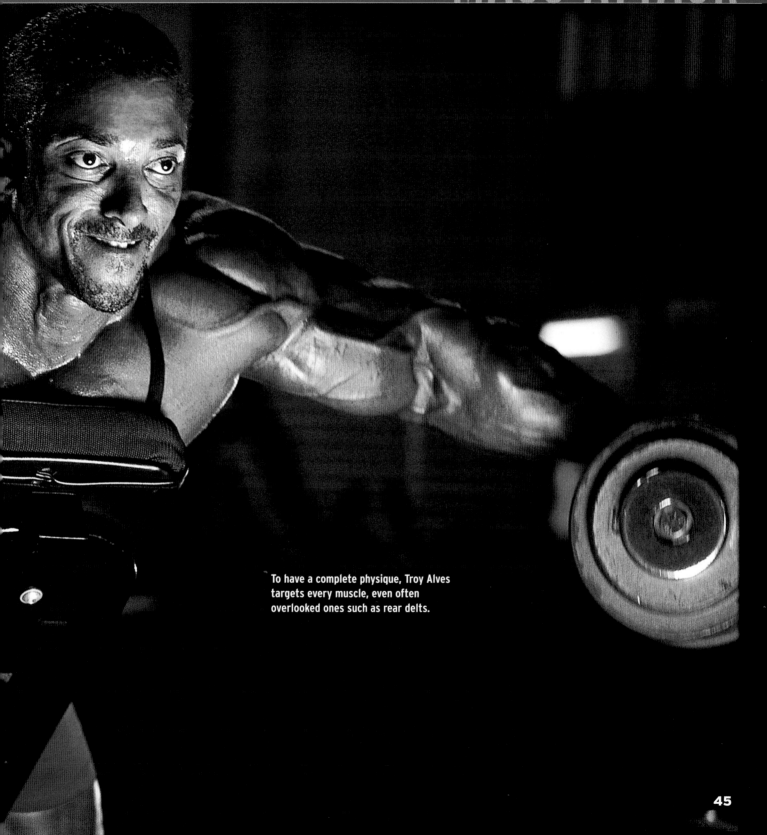

To have a complete physique, Troy Alves targets every muscle, even often overlooked ones such as rear delts.

Dennis Wolf uses lateral raises to develop his middle delt heads.

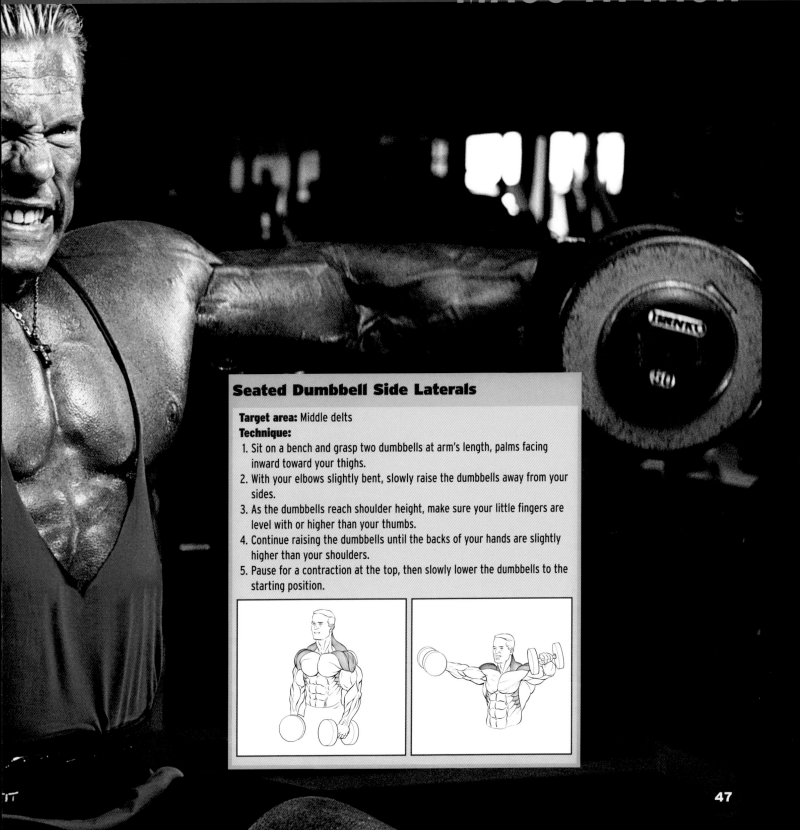

Seated Dumbbell Side Laterals

Target area: Middle delts

Technique:

1. Sit on a bench and grasp two dumbbells at arm's length, palms facing inward toward your thighs.
2. With your elbows slightly bent, slowly raise the dumbbells away from your sides.
3. As the dumbbells reach shoulder height, make sure your little fingers are level with or higher than your thumbs.
4. Continue raising the dumbbells until the backs of your hands are slightly higher than your shoulders.
5. Pause for a contraction at the top, then slowly lower the dumbbells to the starting position.

Performing shrugs and pulldowns helps Garrett Downing develop his upper lats and traps.

Dumbbell Shrugs

Target area: Trapezius
Technique:

1. Hold two dumbbells at arm's length just in front of your body.
2. Keeping your arms straight and using only the power of your traps, shrug your shoulders straight up and hold for a second before slowly returning to the starting position.
3. Do not roll your shoulders back or forward. The shrug should be a straight up and down movement.

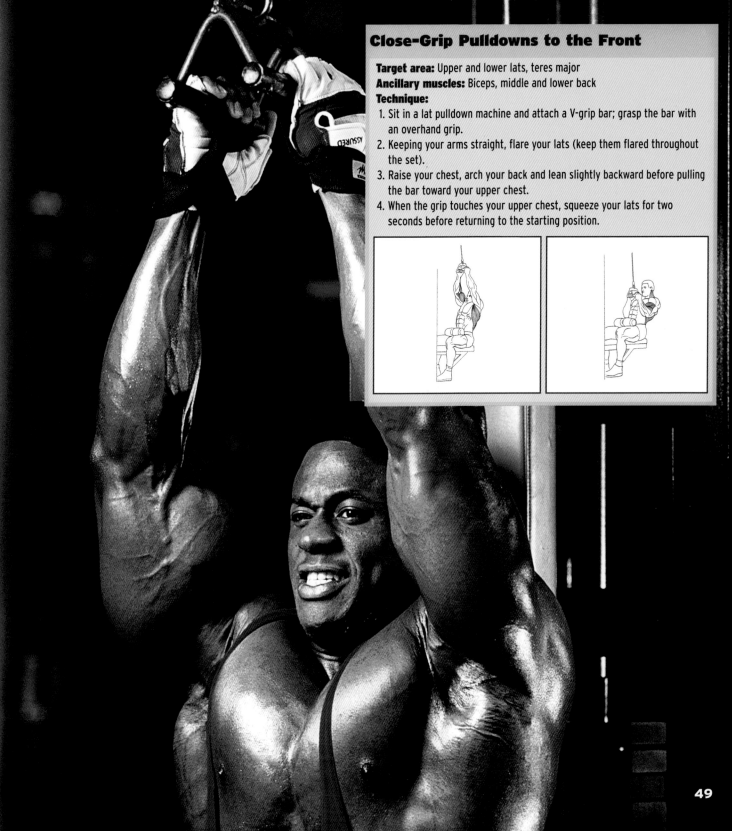

Close-Grip Pulldowns to the Front

Target area: Upper and lower lats, teres major
Ancillary muscles: Biceps, middle and lower back
Technique:

1. Sit in a lat pulldown machine and attach a V-grip bar; grasp the bar with an overhand grip.
2. Keeping your arms straight, flare your lats (keep them flared throughout the set).
3. Raise your chest, arch your back and lean slightly backward before pulling the bar toward your upper chest.
4. When the grip touches your upper chest, squeeze your lats for two seconds before returning to the starting position.

Deadlift

Target area: Lower back
Ancillary muscles: Lats, rhomboids (upper back), glutes, quads
Technique:

1. Assume a balanced stance with feet shoulder width apart.
2. Grasp the bar with your hands spaced just wider than your feet.
3. Bend at the knees while keeping your arms straight and your back flat and straight. Lower your butt until your upper thighs are almost parallel to the floor.
4. Keeping your back flat, slowly straighten your legs—as if you are trying to push your feet through the floor.
5. As the bar reaches knee height, continue to pull the weight upward to put the load on the lower-back muscles.
6. Pull until you are standing upright, with your arms hanging straight. Then roll your shoulders to the rear.
7. Return to the starting position by first bending your legs and then your upper body.

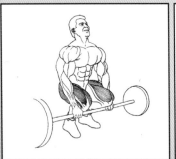 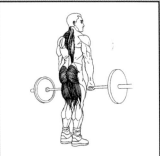

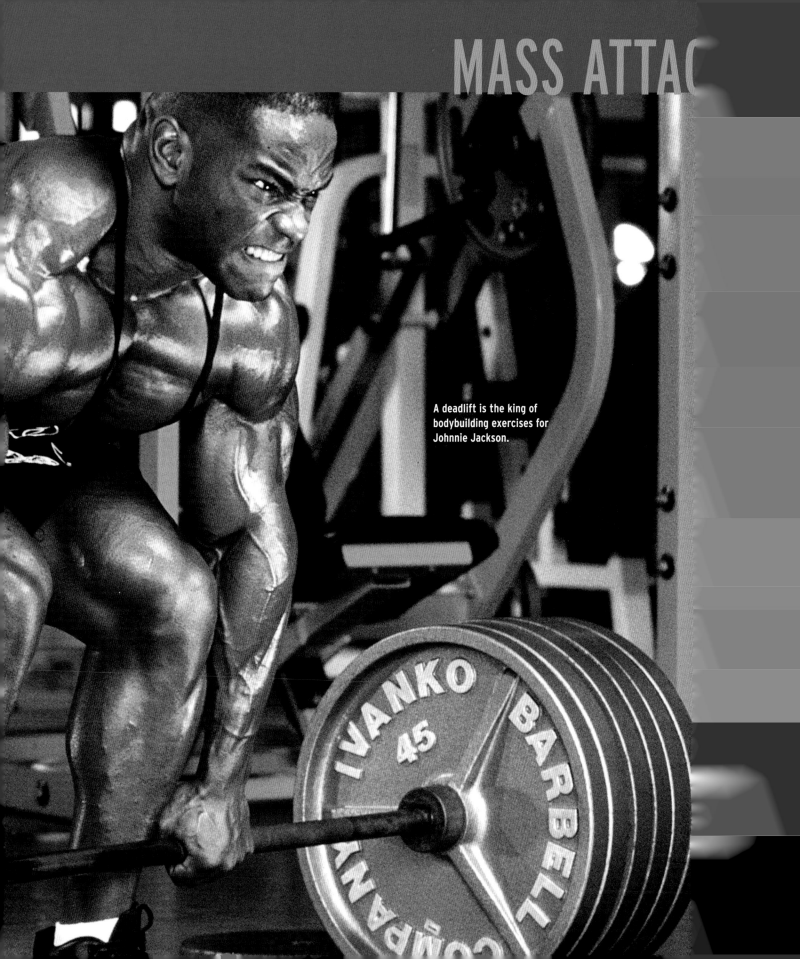

A deadlift is the king of bodybuilding exercises for Johnnie Jackson.

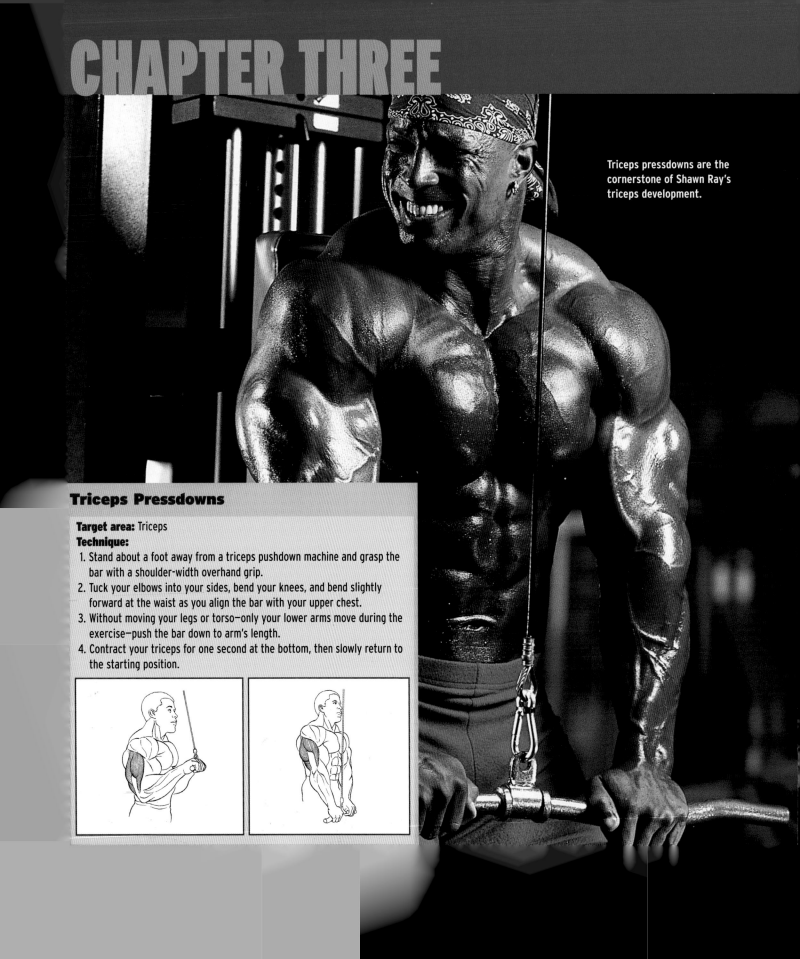

Triceps pressdowns are the cornerstone of Shawn Ray's triceps development.

Triceps Pressdowns

Target area: Triceps

Technique:

1. Stand about a foot away from a triceps pushdown machine and grasp the bar with a shoulder-width overhand grip.
2. Tuck your elbows into your sides, bend your knees, and bend slightly forward at the waist as you align the bar with your upper chest.
3. Without moving your legs or torso—only your lower arms move during the exercise—push the bar down to arm's length.
4. Contract your triceps for one second at the bottom, then slowly return to the starting position.

Incline Dumbbell Curls

Target area: Biceps
Ancillary muscles: Forearms, brachialis
Technique:

1. Sit on an adjustable bench with the back support fixed at a 45-degree angle.
2. Rest your back against the support and grasp two dumbbells, allowing them to hang at arm's length, palms facing each other.
3. While moving only your lower arm, curl the left dumbbell upward. As you approach the point where your elbow joint forms a 90-degree angle, start to turn your wrist while curling. At the top, your palm should face your front delt.
4. From that point, lower the dumbbell, retracing the motion on the way down.
5. As you start the descent with the left dumbbell, begin the ascent-and-rotation phase with the right dumbbell. As the right dumbbell reaches the top, the left one should reach the bottom.

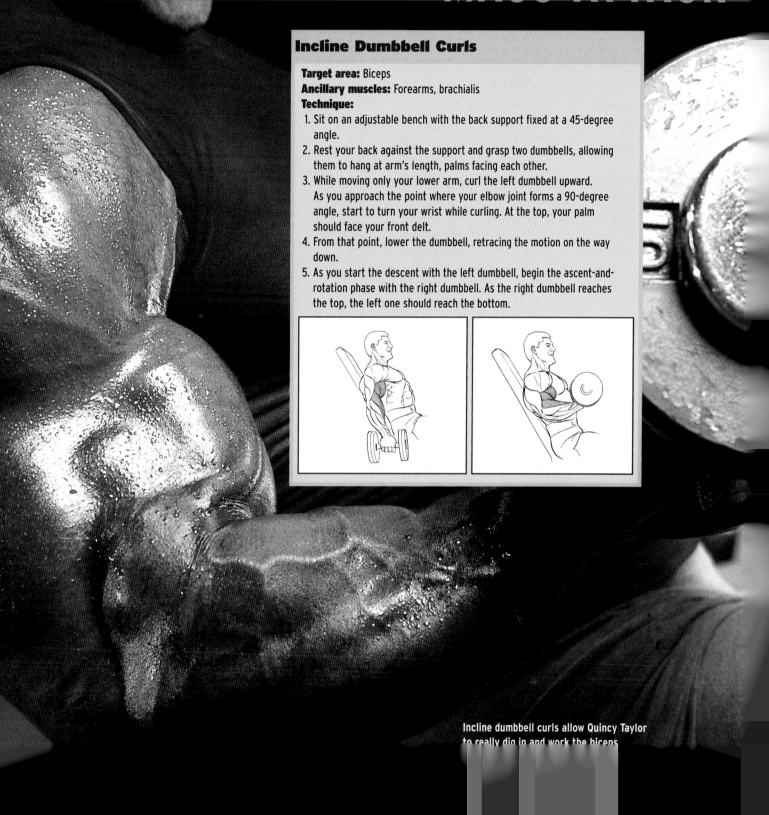

Incline dumbbell curls allow Quincy Taylor to really dig in and work the biceps.

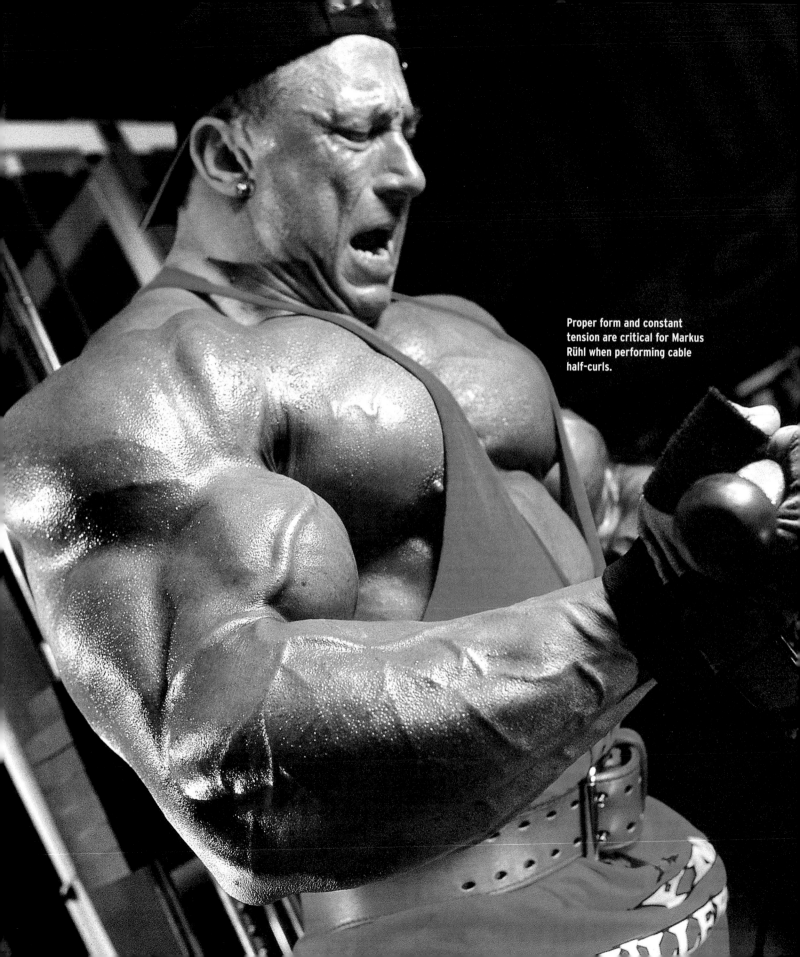

Proper form and constant tension are critical for Markus Rühl when performing cable half-curls.

Perfect FORM

Cultivate bodybuilding's sixth sense to achieve the perfect rep and take your physique to another dimension

It's a deceptively simple question: What is a perfect rep?

From a purely mechanical external view, a rep is the basic unit of bodybuilding. It comprises three phases: positive (or concentric), midpoint (where often a peak contraction is applied) and negative (or eccentric). However, we want you to delve deeper than that; we want you to develop a sixth sense and master the art of executing a perfect rep every time you lift a weight. The true perfect rep comes from within. Like the perfect wave, it has to be felt to be experienced and fully exploited. We're asking you to do something very challenging: Instead of thinking about the mechanics of connecting points A, B and C in performing a rep, we want you to think about feeling and experiencing every rep from within the core of the muscle or muscles being exercised. Perfection, as it applies to reps, calls for a fusion of the physical and mental efforts taking place during your training. Here are the nine fundamentals of achieving the perfect rep.

GET OFF TO A GOOD START

The first step in making the shift from the external to the internal is to make certain that everything you do during every rep is biomechanically correct. This includes your position at the beginning of the set, your performance of the

CHAPTER FOUR

Perfection, as it applies to reps, calls for a fusion of the physical and mental efforts taking place during your training.

first rep and all the reps through to your last one, and your finishing position.

It has been said that it takes 21 days of frequent repetition to create a habit, and many people have spent most of their gym time creating bad habits. By focusing on absolutely perfect biomechanics for three or four weeks, you will etch the proper performance of every rep of every exercise into your subconscious.

2 USE PROPER BODY ALIGNMENT

Many people make a monumental error before they even start their first rep. Without proper body alignment, you are not placing yourself in the optimum position necessary to correctly perform an exercise. In Chapters 2 and 3, we give instructions for the technique required for each exercise in the program. Assume the right posture and biomechanical alignment, then maintain the appropriate parts of your body in that position while you do the work of the set. Stay tight to maximize stability and power.

For instance, for a bench press, it's crucial to start with your shoulders rotated back, shoulder blades pinched together and lats flexed to stabilize the shoulder girdle throughout the movement. If you lift the weight off the rack, thrust your deltoids forward and leave them in that incorrect position throughout the set, you increase the stress on your anterior delts and on the tendons and ligaments of your shoulders. This faulty alignment won't work the pecs hard and, in time, it may lead to a shoulder impingement problem, ultimately making it difficult or painful to bench press.

For standing barbell curls, keep your shoulders rotated back throughout the exercise and keep your midsection tight, with a slight natural arch in your lower back and a slight break in your knees. Visualize pushing through the floor with your heels. This will allow you to safely lift more weight with your biceps. Optimum muscular stress is applied to the targeted area when you maintain proper body alignment.

Cheating techniques may allow you to perform more reps

or use more weight in the short term, but if performed improperly, they will eventually impact your muscle-gaining ability and your success as a bodybuilder. Many inexperienced bodybuilders continue to use improper alignment because they like to feed their egos and pile as much weight on the bar as possible. It may be difficult to swallow your pride and decrease poundages to improve your form. However, optimum muscle gains come only from a platform of proper alignment. Accepting that fundamental change is the first step in moving toward the perfect rep.

3 USE PERFECT FORM

Perfect form is critical to bodybuilding success. No element is more important to bodybuilding than the rep, and no aspect of the rep is more critical than perfect form. By using your muscles as they are built to be used, you are employing the most conducive means of stimulating them to grow. Your challenge is to master the correct biomechanics of the movement and, at the same time, develop a sense of feel in the muscles that enables you to control not only your posture and alignment, but also the areas of the muscles where the stress is greatest.

For instance, when you perform standing barbell curls, make sure your shoulders are rotated back and your upper body is tight with a natural curve to your lower back. Keep your upper arms firmly at your sides as you raise the weight. Contract your glutes and abs to act as stabilizing elements. Maintain this alignment and stay tight for every rep. Many people have a tendency to sway at the waist or raise their upper arms as a way to assist with lifting the weight, but such form breaks put undue stress on the rest of your body and detract from biceps stimulation.

4 DEVELOP THE PROPER MINDSET

Once you have mastered perfect biomechanics, you won't have to think about how to perform a rep or an exercise because your body will have formed that habit. Again, it may

Branch Warren's perfect form and great genes have helped him sculpt world-class calves.

CHAPTER FOUR

Günter Schlierkamp knows that perfect form and inner focus can lead the way to an ultraproductive workout.

take you a month of strict concentration before perfect alignment and form feel natural. When you reach this point, you can begin to move from the external to the internal. You will stop thinking about how to move the weight and begin thinking about how to move your muscles. This is the key to phenomenal gains. This mind shift may be the biggest plateau buster in your workouts.

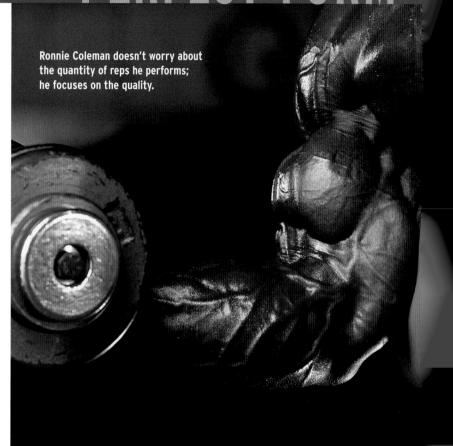

Ronnie Coleman doesn't worry about the quantity of reps he performs; he focuses on the quality.

5 KEEP YOUR MIND FOCUSED ON YOUR TARGET MUSCLES

When you perform any exercise, it's easy to focus on the weight and think about the fact that you're lifting something heavy. That moves you outside your body, though, and focuses your concentration on the external.

Using standing barbell curls as an example again, focus on the stretch and contraction of the biceps. Concentrate on pulling up with your biceps, even if you reach a point where you think you would be able to lift the weight more effectively by recruiting support muscles. Squeeze your biceps at the top, making this an active phase of the rep, instead of resting and regrouping for the next rep.

As you begin to lower the weight, visualize and feel your biceps lengthening. Do this in a controlled fashion to keep the biceps activated throughout the whole rep.

6 MAKE EACH REP COUNT

To get the most from your training, you need to get the most out of each rep. Even in your lightest warm-ups, act as if each rep is a single max attempt. Work the negative for stability and added strength. Often, bodybuilders are so consumed with increasing the number of reps they perform or increasing the amount of weight they lift that they lose sight of their real goal: to add as much muscle mass as possible with the most intense and economical stress.

The rep is at the core of bodybuilding progress. Use as much effort to perform your first rep as you do to perform your last rep. At the beginning of a set, that means putting even more effort into the rep than it actually takes to perform it. Force the target muscle to work as hard as it can, even when that means working it harder than necessary to

complete that rep.

In a perfect world, you should be so focused on each rep that you're unable to count or think past that rep. This is a different mindset than many amateur bodybuilders have, but the pros consistently bring this sharp focus to each rep.

7 DON'T FOCUS ON LIFTING AS MUCH WEIGHT AS POSSIBLE

Maximal muscle growth is not about lifting maximal weight. That's called powerlifting and it's a separate — albeit related — endeavor. The goal of a powerlifter is to lift as much weight as possible. The goal of a bodybuilder is to use as little weight as possible to provide a maximal muscle-building response.

Consider this scenario. Let's say you can bench press 250 pounds for three reps. You have exhausted your pectorals so they cannot lift that weight a fourth time.

If, however, you bench press 225 six times before you are

unable to complete another rep, you have reached a greater threshold of exhaustion. After you have benched 250 three times, you may still be able to bench 225 one time, but after completing six reps at 225, you cannot. Similarly, if you bench 185 for 12 reps before you are unable to press out one more rep, you have reached a still greater level of fatigue.

Of course, you could argue that the greatest fatigue would come from hundreds of reps at a light weight, but that amount would give you diminishing returns as you move from an anaerobic to a more aerobic workout. As a rule of thumb, for your heaviest sets of most exercises, choose a weight that will allow you to successfully complete six to eight reps.

8 AVOID CONSERVATION OF ENERGY

Probably the most common mistake bodybuilders make is to find ways to conserve energy as they perform their reps and sets. When you lock out at the top of a bench press and

To make the most progress, you must apply the optimum muscle stress to the targeted muscle throughout the duration of each set. Rest should come at the end of a set, not in the middle of one.

9 WORK UNTIL YOUR FORM FALTERS

Most bodybuilders have trouble understanding the concept of failure. Clearly, your muscles are going to tire at some point, and you have to be cognizant of that internal sensation so you don't push past the point of maximal benefit and place yourself in the injury zone. Using cheating techniques and energy conservation habits, bodybuilders often try to stave off failure as long as possible, when they would better suit their needs to embrace it.

FLEX defines muscular failure as the point at which you can no longer perform a rep with biomechanically perfect form. Many bodybuilders work past this point, shifting and

Your muscles are going to tire at some point, and you have to be cognizant of that internal sensation so you don't push past the point of maximal benefit and place yourself in the injury zone.

pause (without attempting to perform a muscular contraction), you shift the load off your pectorals and place it on your joints, allowing your pectorals to rest and recover for an instant. You lose intensity and the potential for optimum stress — and full muscle stimulation — to be applied throughout the set.

Many bodybuilders use the negative phase of a rep to rest. This "drop and catch" method means you're not controlling the weight with the appropriate muscle during the negative phase. This is particularly evident in exercises such as bench presses and standing barbell curls, where some bodybuilders allow gravity to perform more of the work than they do.

Bouncing the weight off the chest is another technique for conserving energy during the positive phase of a bench-press rep. This gives the barbell momentum coming off the chest, so you don't have to push the total weight of the bar through a full range of motion. It does not stimulate the pec muscles to their max.

twisting their bodies to get an extra couple of reps. Taking that approach is more likely to lead to injury than to enhanced musculature. When you can no longer lift the weight using your target muscles with perfect form, it's time to stop and prepare for the next set. (Trainers can also use a spotter to help perform one or two more perfect reps after you reach failure.)

GO TO IT

Mastering the perfect rep is both the simplest and most difficult aspect of bodybuilding. By taking this revolutionary approach to focusing on perfecting each rep, you will make profound improvements in your bodybuilding progress. Bodybuilders often focus on external goals as a way of measuring their progress. When you learn to focus on internal goals — intensity and performing the perfect rep — you will advance much more directly toward your long-term bodybuilding goal.

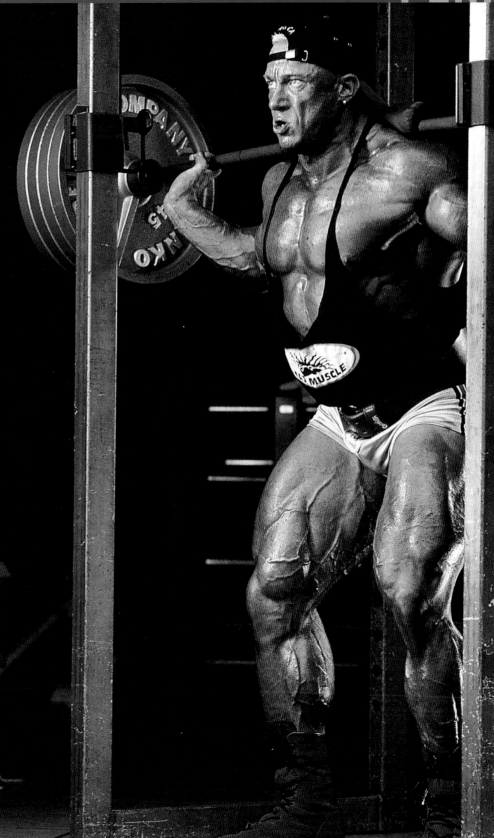

To achieve optimum results,
Rühl squats with textbook form.

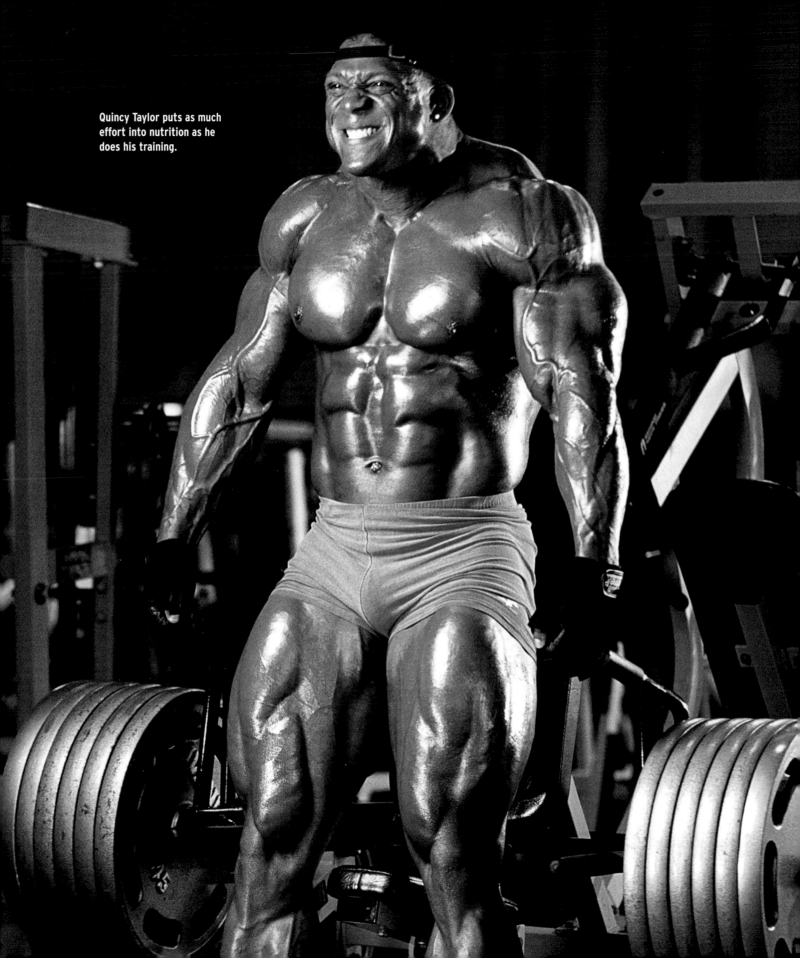

Quincy Taylor puts as much effort into nutrition as he does his training.

The EAT IS ON

Understanding the 10 keys to adding muscle mass

To augment your training, you must eat to get big. Eating for size isn't complicated, as long as you understand it's all a numbers game. If you want to add muscle mass, you have to add calories to your diet. What and how much you eat is the key. In this chapter, we present the 10 crucial components for putting on muscle mass (and an easy key-number method for remembering them), a daily menu guide and a caloric intake chart. Follow these nutrition concepts and, allied with your workouts, you'll develop your muscular potential.

PROTEIN
Key Number: 1

To optimize muscle growth, every bodybuilder should eat at least one gram (g) of protein per pound of bodyweight each day. During a mass-building phase, you can take that up to 1¼ g or more per pound of bodyweight. That means, for instance, a 200-pound bodybuilder should aim to consume 250 g of protein each day.

Protein is the bedrock of the muscle-building process. It is crucial for providing your body with all the amino acids it needs to recover from the stresses of training and hence build muscle mass. In addition, you help prevent muscle breakdown by supplying your body with the extra aminos it needs for other bodily processes and you won't take them from muscle stores.

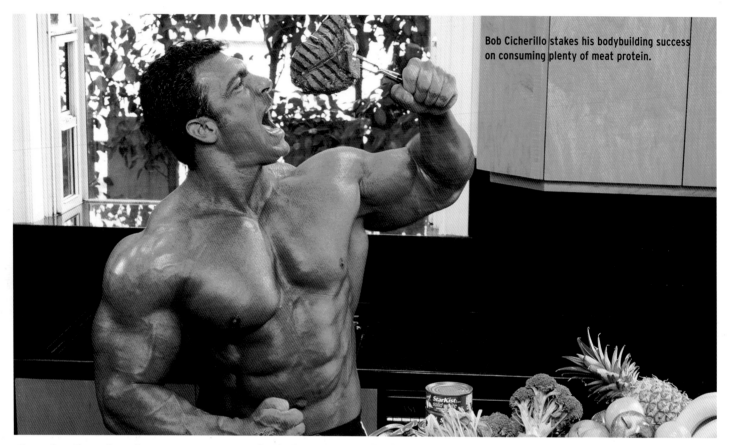

Bob Cicherillo stakes his bodybuilding success on consuming plenty of meat protein.

Carbohydrates are crucial for providing your body with an efficient source of energy to fuel your workouts and add quality mass.

Consuming the proper daily amount of protein is always important for bodybuilders, and it's even easier to accomplish during a mass-building phase because you don't have to be as rigorous with protein food choices. Select chicken and turkey breast, lean red meat, eggs and protein shakes as your fundamental protein foods, but also feel free to eat other cuts of meat, such as lamb, pork, ground beef and dark chicken and turkey meat. These foods are higher in fats, but during a bulking phase, the extra calories can assist your goal of adding quality size.

2 CARBOHYDRATES
Key Numbers: 3-2-1

As in "three to one." Bodybuilders trying to add mass should eat 3 g of carbohydrates per pound of bodyweight every day. Often, bodybuilders get so focused on adding lean mass that they overly restrict the amount of quality carbohydrates they consume, particularly during a mass-building phase. Carbohydrates are crucial for providing your body with an efficient source of energy to fuel your workouts and help you add the quality mass you seek.

During this mass-building phase, a 200-pound bodybuilder would consume approximately 600 g of carbs every day. Fifty to 100 of these should come from simple carbs, such as fruit juice mixed with a postworkout shake or from the sugars in the shake. The remainder should come mostly from complex-carbohydrate foods, such as brown rice, yams, oatmeal, vegetables and high-fiber fruits.

Nasser El Sonbaty consumes carb sources such as pasta to add quality calories to his diet.

Bodybuilders on a mass-building diet can also include starchier carbs, such as white rice, whole-grain breads, white potatoes and pasta, in their daily fare. Starchy carbs are not the ticket during leaning phases, but they are excellent food sources for helping you add muscle mass. Just don't go overboard.

3 FAT
Key Number: 20

Many bodybuilders don't eat enough healthy fats. And bodybuilders with less-than-ideal discipline or insufficient knowledge may eat too much of the wrong types of fat. Ideally, bodybuilders in a mass-building phase should take in 20% of their calories from fats, with two-thirds or more of those coming from healthy fat sources.

To make certain you're getting enough healthy fats, strive to

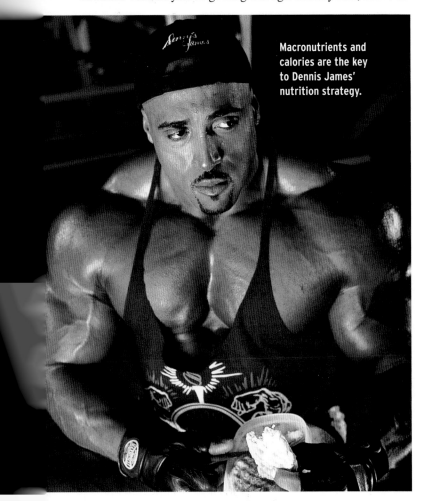

Macronutrients and calories are the key to Dennis James' nutrition strategy.

eat more olives, avocados, fatty fish (e.g., salmon), nuts and seeds, all-natural peanut butter, and olive and canola oil. During a mass-building phase, add oil-based dressings to your salads, plus avocados, olives and walnuts. Eat nuts and seeds as part of your midmorning meal. All-natural peanut butter and a carb-free or low-carb protein shake make for an excellent late-night snack. And, unless you're getting 20-24 ounces of salmon or other fatty cold-water fish a week, be sure to use a flaxseed oil supplement (one to two tablespoons a day).

Overall, you should take in about 60 g of fats on a 3,000-calorie diet and 90 g of fats on a 4,000-calorie diet.

4 CALORIES
Key Number: 33

As in 33%. Calories always count. If you're not getting enough calories, you won't grow, no matter how much you work out or how much attention you place on counting your macronutrients.

Increase calories by a third, and you are providing your body with the additional raw materials it needs to build greater muscle mass. A bodybuilder who consumes roughly 3,000 calories a day for maintenance — about average for a 200-pound bodybuilder — should increase consumption to 4,000 calories daily.

For protein to be retained as muscle mass, you must consume more calories than you need for maintenance. Only those protein calories that are not used for energy or for other bodily functions can be devoted to building new muscle mass. Extra carbohydrates and fats provide readily available energy sources so that protein is accessible for building muscle mass. Carbohydrates then help deliver amino acids to muscles, facilitating the growth process.

5 INCREMENTS
Key Number: 3

Some inexperienced bodybuilders make a massive mistake when trying to increase mass — they add as many calories as possible into their diets as fast as possible. When you begin to bulk up, you're better off doing so in increments.

If your goal is to move from 3,000 calories a day to 4,000 calories a day, do so in three increments of a little more than 300 calories each. After the first bump in intake, maintain that calorie level for about a week to allow your body to adjust. Ultimately, this should help your body use the additional calories more efficiently.

YOUR NUMBERS

All bodybuilders are different from one another, making it hard to be prescriptive about the number of calories any single bodybuilder needs to add muscle mass. One thing is certain, though: You must eat more than what you need for maintenance. Determining how many additional calories you need to add muscle mass comes from experience and learning how your body works. The following chart is designed to give you a starting point on which to base your mass-building diet. Hardgainers may find they need even more calories based on a higher metabolic rate for maintenance.

BODYWEIGHT (IN POUNDS)	125	150	175	200	225
PROTEIN (grams per day)	125-160	150-220	175-250	200-300	225-350
CARBS (grams per day)	375-500	450-550	525-575	600-625	675-725
FAT (grams per day)	60	70	80	90	100
CALORIES (total per day)	3,000	3,400	3,700	4,000	4,500
MEALS (per day)	6-7	6-7	6-7	6-7	6-7

Increase your calories a second time, so you're consuming 3,600 or 3,700 calories a day. Maintain this daily intake level for another week or two, and then take it up a third time to your 4,000-calorie plateau. This total calorie increase of 33% represents an effective bump for most bodybuilders who want to add muscle while adding little bodyfat.

6 MEALS
Key Number: 7

FLEX recommends that bodybuilders eat six meals a day. For those in a bulking phase, seven may prove to be an even more effective number of meals. Simply by adding a protein shake, you can increase your daily consumption by 300 or more calories. If you prefer getting your extra calories from whole foods, spread them among meals throughout the day.

To eat seven meals, you need to get an early start and stick to a schedule. Cramming two or three meals together into one big calorie orgy is less effective than taking in several moderate-sized meals. When you consume 300-1,000 calories (essentially the range for all daily meals, from the smallest to the largest), you distribute calories and energy more evenly throughout the day. If you take in all your calories at once, some are more likely to get stored as bodyfat, even if you're eating the same total number of calories per day.

7 WATER
Key number: 8

You should drink at least eight pints of water per day, and more if you can. Include water when you have protein shakes

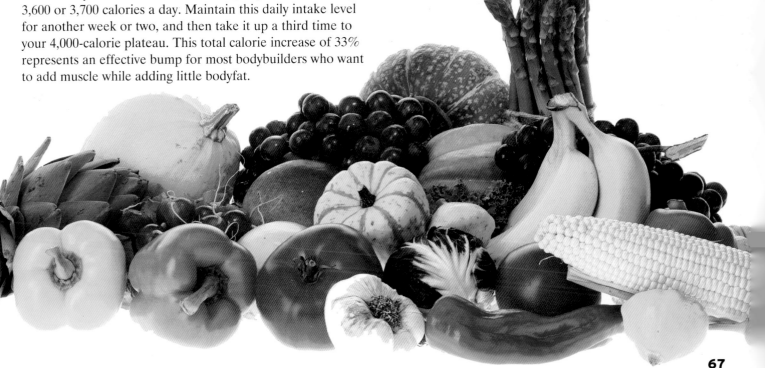

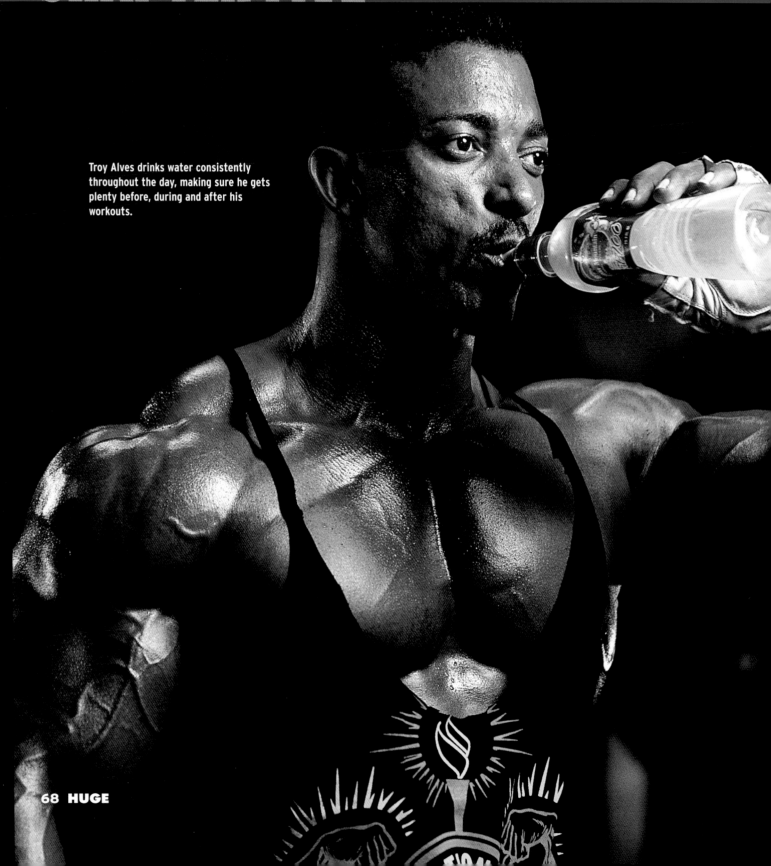

Troy Alves drinks water consistently throughout the day, making sure he gets plenty before, during and after his workouts.

— put in a few more ounces rather than a few less. Drink water between meals and between sets while you're training.

Drinking plenty of water is one of the most overlooked essentials of a bodybuilding diet. Think of it this way: Most bodybuilders seek a muscle pump when they weight train. A muscle pump comes from driving fluid (blood) into your muscles. By keeping yourself well hydrated, you provide your body with what it needs for this simple bodybuilding edge.

And that's only one good reason to keep yourself hydrated. Water is also crucial for flushing toxins from the body and aiding a number of digestive and metabolic processes.

8 FIBER
Key Number: 30

Aim to eat 30 g of fiber per day. Fiber contains no calories, yet it's crucial to a bodybuilding diet, whether you're in a mass-building or cutting phase. Think of fiber as a food processor. It helps your body handle the demands you place on it, whether you're eating a high-protein or a high-calorie diet.

Consume fiber throughout the day. Good sources include oatmeal and whole-grain breads, fruits, vegetables, nuts and seeds. If you aren't consuming 30 g through your diet, strive to do better. You can also add a fiber supplement, such as Metamucil.

If you haven't been taking in 30 g of fiber a day, build up gradually to this amount. Increasing fiber consumption too rapidly can wreak havoc on your digestive system. Add about 2-3 g of fiber every three days or so until you hit your target. This allows your body to incrementally adjust to the increased fiber consumption — the body handles change much better when it occurs gradually.

9 SUPPLEMENTS
Key number: 4

Supplementation can help give you an edge when it comes to adding muscle mass. The four supplements FLEX recommends most enthusiastically are meal-replacement shakes, a multivitamin/multimineral pack, glutamine and creatine.

Meal-replacement shakes provide protein that's easy to digest, plus some carbs and a host of other critical micronutrients. They're excellent for providing an extra meal a day and the additional nutrients you need for muscle growth.

A high-quality multivitamin and multimineral pack contains

BY THE NUMBERS

Here is a quick rundown of the key numbers for getting big and staying big.
- **1** Eat 1 g of protein per pound of bodyweight daily.
- **3** To increase muscle mass while minimizing bodyfat, increase calories in three steps rather than all at once.
- **4** Take these four supplements every day: protein, glutamine, creatine and a multivitamin/multimineral pack.
- **7** Eat seven meals a day during a mass-gaining cycle.
- **8** Drink eight pints of water a day.
- **20** Get 20% of your calories from fat, mostly healthful unsaturated fats.
- **30** Eat 30 g of fiber every day.
- **33** Increase your daily calorie intake by 33% — one-third — in order to sustain muscle growth.
- **3-2-1** Eat quality carbohydrates in a three-to-one ratio of grams to pounds of bodyweight.
- **365** Eat like a bodybuilder consistently 365 days a year.

almost all the micronutrients to ensure that you have no deficiencies in your diet. Take one pack a day. Eating plenty of fruits and vegetables will also help boost your micronutrient levels.

Glutamine is one of the most important muscle-building amino acids. Your body can manufacture glutamine from other aminos, but by supplementing with it, you save your body the effort. In addition, you may spare muscle mass, because to make glutamine, your body pulls aminos from stored muscle mass, which can impact your gains. Take 5-10 g of glutamine twice a day with pre- and posttraining meals.

Creatine, also a combination of amino acids, can help build muscle mass. Taking a small dose of creatine (about 3 g) both before and after a workout will drive fluid into muscles, giving you a greater pump, a better workout and faster recovery.

10 CONSISTENCY
Key number: 365

What's the best way to add muscle mass and keep it? Consistency. Only by adhering to your bodybuilding nutrition plan 365 days a year will you maximize your results. Sure, you'll get good results if you eat properly every other day, but if you want to get ultimate bodybuilding results, you have to eat like a bodybuilder every day of your life.

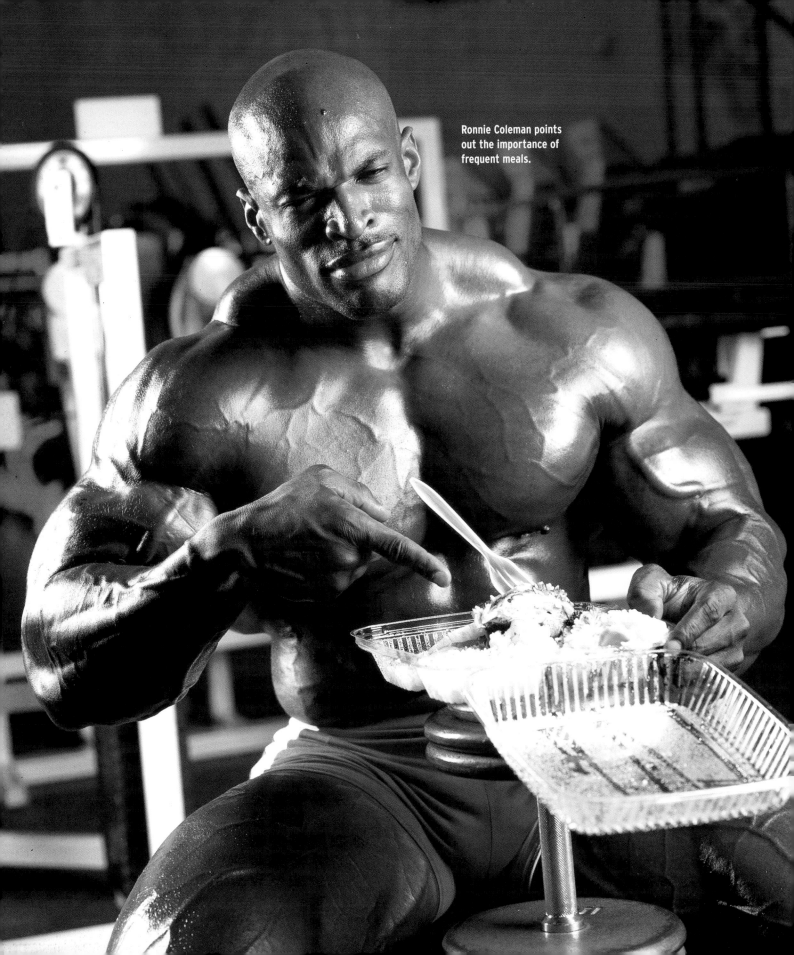

Ronnie Coleman points out the importance of frequent meals.

Feeding the FURNACE

Use these meal plans to add 10 pounds of muscle in three to six months.

Increasing muscle mass without adding significant physique-obscuring bodyfat requires a rigorous program. *FLEX* has laid out two basic plans: One is designed to help you add 10 pounds of muscle mass in three months without significantly increasing bodyfat; the other allows you to accomplish the same goal over six months. It may seem like a no-brainer. Who wouldn't want to add 10 pounds of muscle in three months, rather than six? The answer has much more to do with you and your lifestyle than with the intensity of your desire

for more muscle mass. The three-month plan is very demanding; the six-month plan is more accommodating of other segments of your life. How do you know which plan is right for you? Read on, and we'll help you choose.

Part 1: Pick Your Plan

In general, increasing muscle mass without adding bodyfat is more easily done over longer time periods with consistency, but if circumstances are in your favor, it can be done quickly with strict discipline. The best time to add muscle mass is when you are under relatively low stress and you have the time to recuperate and grow. Perhaps you've noticed in the past that you tend to increase your muscle mass in relatively short spurts, even when you follow a consistent long-term program. Two factors come into play: variables you can control and those you can't.

Aside from dedication, discipline and hard work, you must also outline bodybuilding goals that are achievable. If your goals are unreasonable, then you've set yourself up for failure. Knowing what your body (and schedule) are capable of can help you establish aims that you can reasonably expect to achieve. We've listed some physical and lifestyle characteristics that will help you determine whether a shorter or longer muscle-gaining plan is better for you.

THREE-MONTH PLAN If you fit into any of the categories below, you might reasonably expect to be able to add 10 pounds of muscle mass in three months.

Bodybuilders — old or young — trying to add muscle mass for the first time If you're a beginning or a less-experienced bodybuilder trying to add 10 pounds of new muscle mass, then you may be able to do so relatively quickly, since your body is unaccustomed to the rigors of weight training and will be shocked into growth.

Bodybuilders who have neglected their nutrition If you have been training regularly, but haven't put much effort or thought into your nutrition, then you may be a prime candidate to make amazing gains when you start a solid (and new for you) nutrition program geared to muscle gains.

Bodybuilders who have taken a long break from training If you've taken off training for a while, you might note astounding results when you return to the gym.

Bodybuilders ready for a growth phase Is your body primed for a growth phase? There's no way to tell other than to go on this program. Our body rhythms are cyclical, but many people tend to make size gains quickly. This might be that time for you. If not, allow your body the luxury of more time to grow — try the six-month program.

SIX-MONTH PLAN Trainers who don't fit into any of the earlier categories may find it challenging to add 10 pounds of muscle mass in a short period of time without significantly increasing bodyfat. Keep in mind that most experienced bodybuilders rarely add more than 10 pounds of muscle mass in a year. To do so in six months is still an amazing accomplishment and a more realistic expectation for bodybuilders who fall into one of the following categories.

Bodybuilders who have been consistent with their training and nutrition If your nutrition and training programs are already pretty good, you can't make as great a comparative improvement as someone who has nutrition or training deficiencies. That may seem unfair, but keep in mind that you've probably already added 10 (or 20 or 30) pounds of muscle mass that they're trying to add. For you to add yet another 10 pounds of muscle mass, you're going to have to apply even more discipline, and you're probably going to have to do it gradually.

Bodybuilders who have busy lifestyles that often interrupt their nutritional and training demands Many successful bodybuilders have had to make difficult choices, prioritizing their training and nutrition ahead of family, friends, education or career advancement. If you're able to devote yourself only part-time to bodybuilding, you can still make phenomenal gains, albeit more slowly.

Bodybuilders who are endomorphs Endomorphs (bigger guys

If you want to add muscle mass, you must add calories, regardless of whether your plan is to add that muscle quickly or more slowly.

with a tendency toward being overweight) are predisposed to putting on bodyfat more easily than their ecto- and mesomorphic counterparts. Increasing calories 20-30%, as both plans recommend, can be a sure-fire way to pack on fat pounds as well as muscle. Many endomorphs need to increase calories just slightly (about 10% above baseline) in order to add muscle at a pace that limits bodyfat accumulation. For this group, the six-month plan is a more viable option.

Part 2: Getting Prepped

If you want to add muscle mass, you must add calories, regardless of whether your plan is to add that muscle quickly or more slowly. Increasing calories can be more challenging than it seems — it's not always simply a matter of eating more food. It's a matter of eating the right foods at the right times and in the right quantities.

One of the best ways to increase calories is to carefully calculate the amount of food you eat for maintenance.

Shawn Ray says you can shrug as much as you want, but you need to be decisive in choosing your plan.

That's your baseline. Making this calculation may seem tedious, but it's the most effective way to establish your nutritional requirements.

KEEP A FOOD LOG Keep a food diary of everything you eat and drink and the amounts you take in for a whole week before you start your new program. One of your greatest challenges is to keep an accurate record of what you eat without changing your consumption habits in anticipation of your diet. In other words, avoid making any changes during the first seven days.

Write down all the foods you eat. Keep your meal frequency and food selection as close as possible to your norm. Weigh or measure portion sizes as accurately as possible (a small high-quality scale is a valuable tool for this serious dietary program) so that you can make accurate calculations of calories and macronutrients.

Check out our chart on calories and macronutrients of select bodybuilding foods on page 87. For more comprehensive listings, *FLEX* recommends *The Complete Book of Food Counts* by Corinne T. Netzer, as well as the U.S. Department of Agriculture's nutrient database Web site at www.nal.usda.gov/fnic/ foodcomp/search.

CAREFULLY ASSESS YOUR PHYSIQUE
You have to be impartial and nonjudgmental for this to be effective. We recommend that you take pictures of yourself at various stages of the diet so you can be objective — and accurate — about your physique changes. Also, have a friend scrutinize you (and vice versa, if you are on the diet together).

Part 3: Beginning Your Nutrition Program
THE THREE-MONTH PLAN EXPLAINED
The biggest challenge is to eat all the quality foods in the

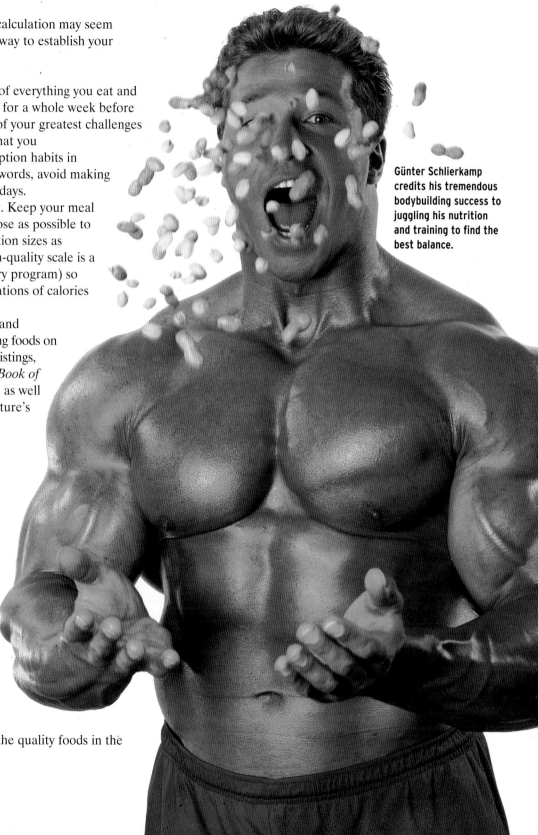

Günter Schlierkamp credits his tremendous bodybuilding success to juggling his nutrition and training to find the best balance.

quantity that you need to make gains. Implement these phases as soon as you have completed your weeklong food log to calculate your daily caloric baseline.

Phase One: Days 1-10 On each of these days, you'll augment your baseline diet by 300-500 calories daily. To compute how much you should add, follow these broad-based recommendations. All bodybuilders should increase consumption by 300 calories. Those who normally eat 3,000 or more calories a day for maintenance should add another 100 calories per day. Those who consider themselves to be hardgainers should consume an additional 100 calories per day beyond that. (Hardgainers who eat 3,000 calories a day for maintenance should take in 3,000 + 300 + 100 + 100 = 3,500 total calories per day.)

By eating 300 to 500 more calories a day during this first phase, you allow your body to gradually accommodate to an increased nutritional level. Continue to keep your food log, and check your numbers to make certain you're eating as much as you think you are.

Note that the meal plans accompanying this chapter list intakes of 3,700-3,900 calories daily. If your requirements are lower (as for a bodybuilder who requires fewer than 3,000 baseline calories per day for maintenance), reduce some of the suggested quantities of foods slightly. Try to lower protein and complex carbohydrate consumption equally. For example, eat slightly less oatmeal, eat one less egg in the morning, reduce meat portions slightly for your evening meal, and eat a smaller baked potato. By making three or four small adjustments, you can easily adapt the 3,700- to 3,900-calorie daily meal plans so you're taking in 3,300-3,500 calories daily. Eat six meals a day, regardless of your level of calorie consumption.

After 10 days, carefully evaluate your physique in a mirror. Does it appear that you're adding bodyfat? It shouldn't. You should be fuller, harder, heavier and stronger. If you appear to be adding more bodyfat, take the longer (six-month) approach to adding muscle mass.

Phase Two: Days 11-21: During this stage, most bodybuilders should add another 300-500 calories daily, totaling 600-1,000 calories more than needed for maintenance. Use the same formula as in phase one to determine your needs. (Everyone adds at least 300 calories; hardgainers add 100 more to that amount; and those who normally take in at least 3,000 for maintenance consume an additional 100 calories.) Bodybuilders who noticed increases in bodyfat levels after

BASIC BODYBUILDING FOODS

In the accompanying table, we list many of the most basic bodybuilding foods, their protein and carbohydrate content in grams (g) for suggested serving sizes, and their calorie counts. Use this chart in two ways: first, to compute your baseline calorie consumption before you start the add-mass program; second, to choose food substitutions for your daily meal plans once you begin the diet.

FOOD (SERVING SIZE)	PROTEIN (G)	CARBS (G)	CALORIES
Almonds (2 oz)	12	10	340
Avocado (2 oz)	1	4	100
Banana (1 medium)	1	28	110
Beans/lentils (4 oz dry)	21	54	300
Berries (4 oz)	0	11	50
Bread (2 slices whole grain)	12	48	240
Cheese (4 oz low fat)	36	4	320
Chicken (6 oz canned)	33	0	150
Chicken breast (8 oz skinless)	48	0	360
Cottage cheese (1 cup low fat)	30	7	190
Eggs (6 whole)	38	3	450
Egg whites (12)	42	3	200
Fish (8 oz lean, white)	43	0	210
Ground beef (8 oz extra lean)	40	0	600
Milk (1 quart nonfat)	36	48	360
Oatmeal (100 g dry)	14	60	330
Olive oil (1 tbsp)	0	0	120
Orange (1 medium)	1	16	65
Pasta (6 oz)	21	120	630
Peanut butter (6 tbsp commercial)	21	18	570
Peanut butter (6 tbsp natural)	30	15	600
Peanuts (2 oz)	14	12	320
Potato, baked (5" x 2", with skin)	5	50	220
Potato, baked (8 oz, no skin)	4	50	210
Rice (½ cup precooked, brown)	10	70	320
Rice (½ cup precooked, white)	6	70	320
Salmon (8 oz Atlantic)	45	0	420
Sardines (6 oz in oil, drained)	45	0	360
Spinach (8 oz frozen)	6	6	50
Steak (8 oz New York)	62	0	500
Steak (8 oz round)	66	0	430
Tuna (6 oz canned)	33	0	150
Turkey bacon (4 oz)	22	0	150
Turkey breast (8 oz)	65	0	430
Vegetables (6 oz frozen, mixed)	4	10	60
Yams (8 oz baked)	2	38	160
Yogurt (8 oz plain)	13	17	120

In putting on muscle mass, Coleman says you can do it quickly or in shades.

For both plans, you'll essentially "overeat" nutritious foods that help stimulate muscle growth.

phase one shouldn't add calories during phase two.

After 21 days on this dietary program, again carefully evaluate your physique to determine if you are adding too much bodyfat. If you are, scale back on your food consumption, reducing carbohydrate calories rather than fats or protein. If you are pleased with your progress, continue to eat this quantity of food on a daily basis as you move into phase three.

Phase Three: Days 22-90 The first day of every week, starting with day 22, should be a higher carb day. Increase complex carbs from the best sources, such as yams, brown rice and oatmeal, taking in approximately 200 extra calories (50 g of carbohydrates) from these foods spread out over the first four meals of the day. However, don't increase calories much — reduce protein and fat consumption somewhat to keep from driving total calorie consumption too high.

If you are content with your bodyfat levels, you can eat higher carbs twice a week. (See "Carbohydrate Intake" on page 90.) But don't overdo it — consuming more carbs once or twice a week may help promote muscle building in the presence of training and protein, but overeating carbs can lead to greater bodyfat storage. Keep a careful watch on your physique so you can make dietary adjustments and avoid adding too much bodyfat.

If you need to reduce bodyfat, drop 200 calories worth of carbs two to four days a week. If you believe your body has accommodated to the three weekly 30-minute cardio sessions you'll be doing for this program, then increase those sessions to 40 minutes each. Keep them at three times a week, though, as performing too much cardio can undermine muscle gains.

THE SIX-MONTH PLAN EXPLAINED

The biggest difference between the three- and six-month plans is that you don't need to be as intense to add 10 pounds of muscle over the longer time period. For both plans, you'll essentially "overeat" nutritious foods that help stimulate muscle growth. The longer program, though, doesn't require you to be as rigorous with each day's nutrition plan. The six-month plan still requires discipline, but it permits you to include "cheat days," allowing you to eat nutritious but less-than-ideal bodybuilding foods, such as lasagna, hamburgers and pizza.

By adhering rigorously to your diet five days a week, allowing for one cheat day and perhaps another of unintentional undereating or dietary straying, you can still make progress, as long as you stay devoted to your long-range goals. This is a much more usable plan for those with busy lifestyles who want to make bodybuilding gains, but feel they can't make it the central focus of their lives 24/7.

Phase One: Days 1-10 This is the same as for the three-month plan — increase calories by 300-500 per day.

Phase Two: Days 11-20 This is also the same as for the three-month plan. Increase calories by another 300-500 daily. (Based on a 3,000-calorie baseline for bodyweight maintenance, a trainer would be eating 3,600-4,000 total calories per day at this point.)

Phase Three: Days 21-180 Phase three of the six-month plan differs from that of the three-month version in the following ways.

- You eat about the same amount of calories each day, but take in slightly more calories from carbohydrates.

- It includes one cheat day a week. On that day, follow your bodybuilding diet for the most part, but you can incorporate a cheat food or two and a cheat meal. The best bodybuilding cheat foods are high in protein (pizza and hamburgers) rather than just high in calories (doughnuts, sodas and French fries). Keep this in mind as you make your food choices. Cheat foods allow more than just a psychological break — they can help you fill out and recover from the rigors of training and dieting. But they do increase the risk of storing bodyfat.

- It also allows a cheat food, if you want, on one other day a week.

- It requires you to evaluate whether you need to make shifts in your diet. If you believe you are overdieted, include a "recharge" week, during which you modify the basic plan of the diet. (See "Weekly Carbohydrate Strategies.")

Continue to evaluate your physique every seven to 10 days to determine whether you need to make shifts in your diet, either in terms of total calories or in macronutrient ratios.

Part 4: Putting it All Together With Meal Plans

In both the three- and six-month plans, eat approximately 20-30% more calories per day than needed for baseline body-weight management. At the same time, keep carbohydrates relatively low, but high enough to avoid feeling and looking depleted. To prevent bodyfat storage, vary the amount of carbohydrates you take in on a daily basis. We provide you with carbohydrate strategies for the three- and six-month plans, plus two others designed for specific purposes, as well as sample meal plans to put these strategies into practice.

WEEKLY CARBOHYDRATE STRATEGIES

The following weekly strategies create "metabolic confusion," helping to prevent your body from storing excess calories as bodyfat. Altering carb intake from day to day encourages your body to burn calories and stored bodyfat, rather than increasing fat storage. Your total bodyweight should increase through the addition of muscle mass, not bodyfat.

The number of carbohydrates you should take in to promote growth without accumulating significant amounts

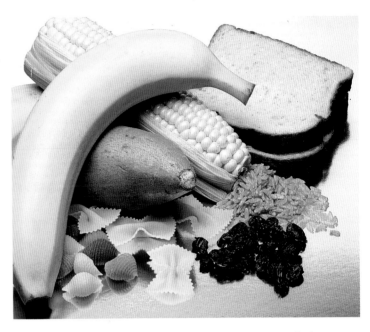

of bodyfat is individual. As such, these recommendations are averages. They may be ideal for you, or you may need to make changes as you see the effects they have on your physique.

Altering carb intake from day to day encourages your body to burn calories and stored bodyfat.

SAMPLE MEAL PLANS

The four meal plans in this chapter offer examples of the types of daily nutrition plans you might put together for your add-mass program. Each meal plan offers a different total carb count per day — from 250-400 g. The goal is to keep close track of the amount of carbs you take in every day, while allowing for all the protein and calories needed for muscular growth.

Each daily meal plan has 3,700-3,900 calories and 320-350 g of protein. FLEX established these baselines as averages our readers will need for success. If you find that you need to consume fewer or more calories than these meals provide, eat the same foods and the same number of meals, but reduce or increase portion sizes across the board. This will keep your

CARBOHYDRATE INTAKE

	THREE-MONTH PLAN	SIX-MONTH PLAN	VARIETY	RECHARGE
Monday	250	250	250	Cheat
Tuesday	250	250	300	400
Wednesday	250	350	350	400
Thursday	300	250	Cheat	350
Friday	250	250	250	250
Saturday	250	Cheat	250	350
Sunday	400	300	400	250

See the sample meal plans elsewhere in this chapter to help you achieve these daily carb counts.

Notes: The goal of the three-month plan is to help you add 10 pounds of muscle mass quickly while putting on little bodyfat. On this plan, eat a reduced amount of carbohydrates, but still enough to allow for muscle growth under ideal circumstances. On the six-month plan, consume a slightly higher carbohydrate count than on the three-month plan. Hardgainers or people with a fast metabolism may choose to use this time frame for adding muscle mass. For variety, you may choose, after three or four weeks on either of the basic plans, to help your progress along by taking in a few more carbs over the course of a week. This may help amp up metabolic confusion. Recharge by infusing your diet with a week of higher carbs if you feel overtrained, if you have trouble recovering from training, or if you feel weak after following the other comparatively low-carb plans.

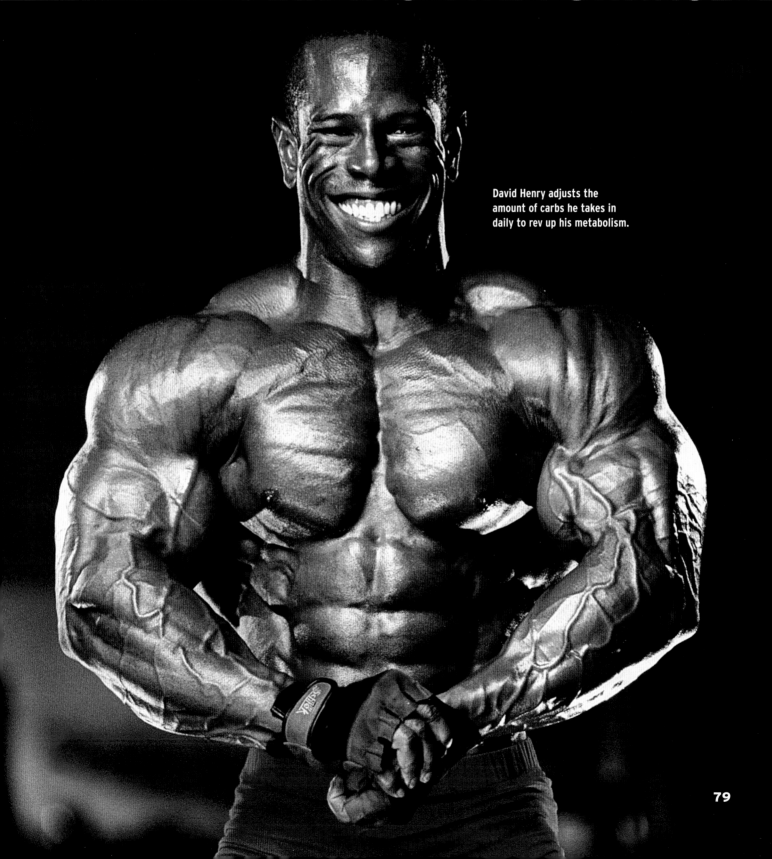

David Henry adjusts the amount of carbs he takes in daily to rev up his metabolism.

MEAL PLAN 1: 250 G OF CARBS PER DAY

	Calories	Protein	Carbs
Meal one, 7 AM (breakfast)			
6 large eggs	450	38	3
4 oz turkey bacon	150	22	0
50 g oatmeal	165	7	30
Piece of fruit	65	1	17
Meal two, 10 AM (snack)			
4 tbsp natural peanut butter	400	20	10
1 slice whole-grain bread	120	6	24
Meal three, 1 PM (lunch)			
8 oz skinless chicken breast	360	48	0
2 slices whole-grain bread	240	12	48
2 oz avocado	100	1	4
Meal four, 3 PM (preworkout)			
8 oz low-fat cottage cheese	190	30	7
Meal five, 6 PM and 7 PM (postworkout)			
Immediately after training			
Postworkout drink	320	40	40
About an hour later			
8 oz extra-lean hamburger	580	57	0
8 oz baked potato (no skin)	210	4	50
5 oz broccoli	50	4	8
Meal six, 9 PM			
Whey protein powder drink	200	50	0
2 tbsp natural peanut butter	200	10	5
TOTALS (APPROXIMATE)	**3,800**	**350**	**250**

MEAL PLAN 2: 300 G OF CARBS PER DAY

	Calories	Protein	Carbs
Meal one, 7 AM (breakfast)			
6 large eggs	450	38	3
100 g oatmeal	330	14	60
Piece of fruit	65	1	17
Meal two, 10 AM (snack)			
4 oz turkey breast	220	32	0
2 slices whole-grain bread	240	12	48
Meal three, 1 PM (lunch)			
8 oz skinless chicken breast	360	48	0
½ cup (precooked) brown rice	320	10	70
2 oz avocado	100	1	4
Meal four, 3 PM (preworkout)			
8 oz low-fat cottage cheese	190	30	7
Meal five, 6 PM and 7 PM (postworkout)			
Immediately after training			
Postworkout drink	320	40	40
About an hour later			
8 oz New York steak	500	62	0
8 oz baked yams	160	2	38
5 oz broccoli	50	4	8
Meal six, 9 PM			
Whey protein powder drink	200	50	0
2 tbsp natural peanut butter	200	10	5
TOTALS (APPROXIMATE)	**3,700**	**350**	**300**

To build an eye-catching six-pack in the style of Ahmad Haidar, you have to pack in the right amount of carbs each day.

MEAL PLAN 3: 350 G OF CARBS PER DAY

	Calories	Protein	Carbs
Meal one, 7 AM (breakfast)			
6 large eggs	450	38	3
100 g oatmeal	330	14	60
Meal two, 10 AM (snack)			
4 oz turkey breast	220	32	0
2 slices whole-grain bread	240	12	48
Meal three, 1 PM (lunch)			
8 oz Atlantic salmon	420	42	0
½ cup (precooked) brown rice	320	10	70
6 oz mixed frozen vegetables	60	4	10
Meal four, 3 PM (preworkout)			
8 oz low-fat cottage cheese	190	30	7
Meal five, 6 PM and 7 PM (postworkout)			
Immediately after training			
Get-big drink	600	40	100
About an hour later			
8 oz New York steak	500	62	0
5" x 2" baked potato with skin	220	5	50
8 oz frozen spinach	50	6	6
Meal six, 9 PM			
Whey protein powder drink	200	50	0
TOTALS (APPROXIMATE)	**3,800**	**340**	**350**

MEAL PLAN 4: 400 G OF CARBS PER DAY

	Calories	Protein	Carbs
Meal one, 7 AM (breakfast)			
6 large eggs	450	38	3
100 g oatmeal	330	14	60
Meal two, 10 AM (snack)			
4 oz turkey breast	220	32	0
2 slices whole-grain bread	240	12	48
Meal three, 1 PM (lunch)			
8 oz Atlantic salmon	420	42	0
½ cup (precooked) brown rice	320	10	70
Meal four, 3 PM (preworkout)			
32 oz nonfat milk	360	36	48
Meal five, 6 PM and 7 PM (postworkout)			
Immediately after training			
Get-big drink (½ serving)	300	20	50
About an hour later			
8 oz skinless chicken breast	360	48	0
6 oz pasta	630	21	120
5 oz broccoli	50	4	8
Meal six, 9 PM			
Whey protein powder drink	200	50	0
TOTALS (APPROXIMATE)	**3,900**	**320**	**400**

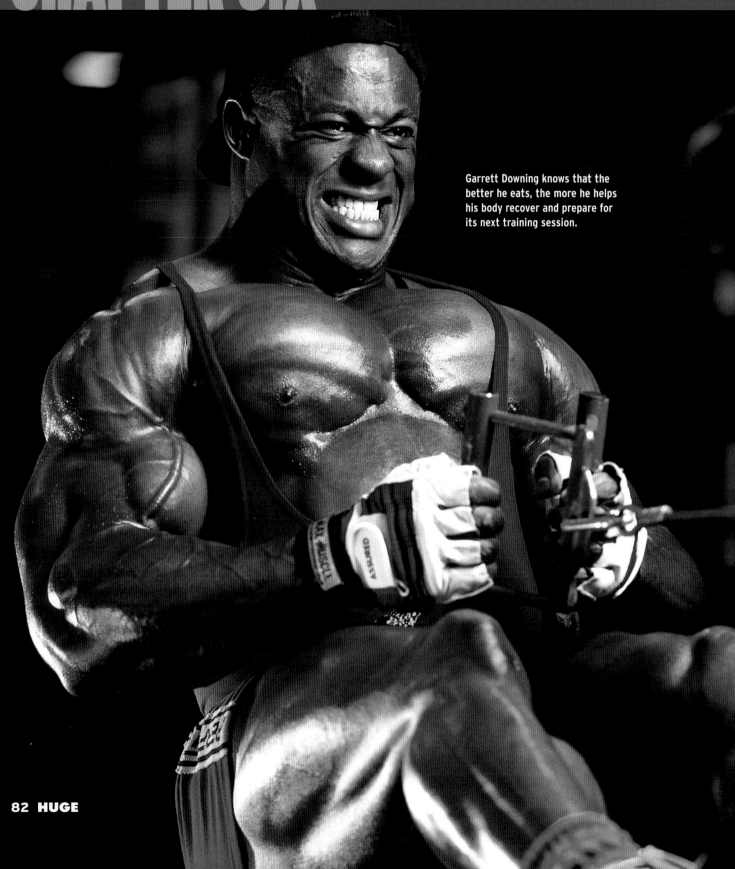

Garrett Downing knows that the better he eats, the more he helps his body recover and prepare for its next training session.

Good planning and psychological preparation are key to any successful diet.

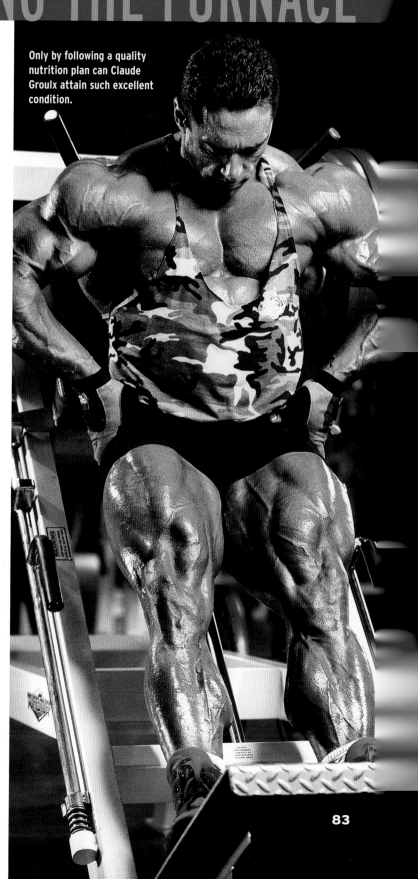

Only by following a quality nutrition plan can Claude Groulx attain such excellent condition.

macronutrient ratios the same while allowing you to make the necessary calorie adjustments.

Part 5: Diet Strategies

Good planning and psychological preparation are key to any successful diet. Two factors that can quickly sabotage a bodybuilding diet are missing meals and stressing over missed meals. Follow these tips to avoid those situations.

1. STRICTLY ADHERE TO YOUR DIET AT ALL TIMES.

Bring as much discipline to your diet as you bring to weight training. Build your days around your nutrition program and follow through.

2. DON'T STRESS IF YOU MISS A MEAL.

On occasion, circumstances may cause you to miss a meal or to eat foods that are less than ideal. When that happens, getting stressed out will do much more harm to your physique than the missed meal itself.

3. PREPARE FOR PROBLEMS.

Always carry a few ready-to-eat meals in a cooler. You never know when you might be delayed at work or school.

4. EAT MORE FOOD EARLIER IN THE DAY.

If you have concerns that you won't be able to consume all the meals and quantities of foods that your diet calls for, use early meals to make up the difference. Add a third morning meal or eat slightly more food at your first two meals of the day.

5. KEEP CARBS MODERATE.

Once you've established your daily plan, watch your carb intake to make certain that you are taking in the proper amount for that day. Eating too few carbs will dramatically undercut your ability to add muscle mass. Eating too many will add more bodyfat than you want.

6. EVALUATE THE PLAN AND ADAPT IT TO YOUR NEEDS.

Never forget that this is your diet plan, and that you are ultimately responsible for all aspects of it. That gives you the freedom to make any adaptations you deem suitable for your body.

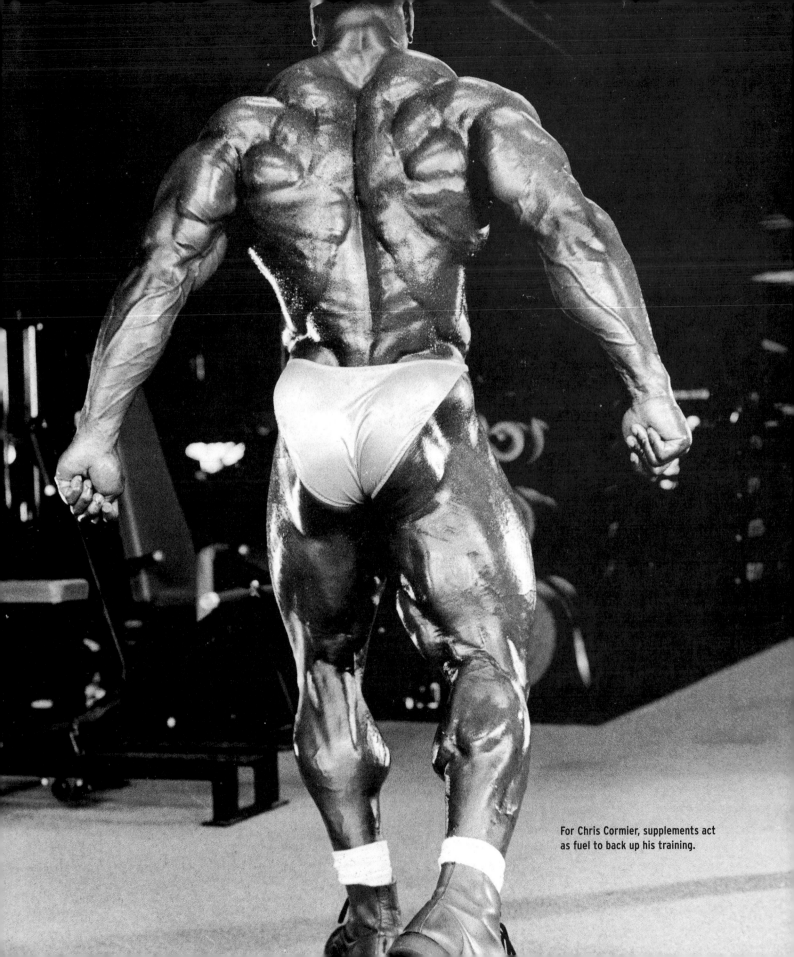

For Chris Cormier, supplements act as fuel to back up his training.

Bodybuilding BOOSTERS

Make basic gains or achieve specific goals with the right supplements

Supplementation is a key aspect of bodybuilding, but we've held off discussing it in detail until this chapter for a very good reason: It's important to put supplementation into perspective. You can make bodybuilding gains without supplementation. However, you cannot make bodybuilding gains without proper training and nutrition; the first few chapters of this book have focused almost exclusively on those cornerstones.

Supplementation enhances and promotes the gains derived from training and nutrition. Too much emphasis on supplementation sends the message that consuming powders, pills and drinks — in the absence of proper training and nutrition — will provide the muscle growth you seek. If you over-emphasize supplementation, you might even begin to slack off on your training and basic nutrition. Being mindful of those caveats, you can use the basic supplements recommended here to get more out of your training and nutrition, and you can take the specialty supplements to help you overcome certain stumbling blocks or achieve specific objectives.

THE BASICS
Whether you're taking supplements already, or you never

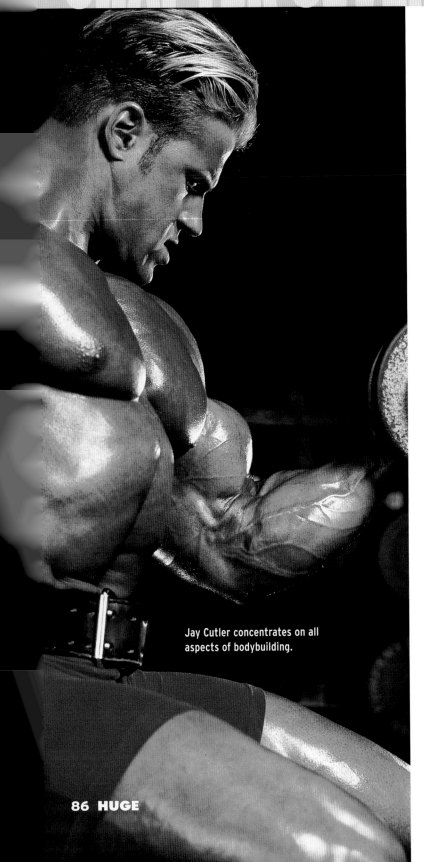

Jay Cutler concentrates on all aspects of bodybuilding.

have before, read through our list of recommendations to see what's right for you.

PROTEIN To build muscle mass, you must supply your body with the necessary amino acids found in protein. For this reason, given an overall adequate diet, protein consumption is the single most important factor of bodybuilding nutrition, so it's not surprising that it's also one of the critical aspects of supplementation. Often, it's hard (and expensive) for bodybuilders to take in all the protein from food that they need for building muscle. Supplementing with protein in the form of premixed drinks or shakes made from powder can supply your daily needs.

Recommendation: Consume at least 1 gram (g) of protein per pound of bodyweight every day, from supplements and from whole foods. On balance, strive to get as much protein as possible from your food. As a rule of thumb, you might supplement with a drink that contains whey and simple carbs

The most prevalent free amino acid in muscle, glutamine is necessary for many vital physiological functions.

(30-50 g of protein) taken after training, and one protein shake without carbs (30-50 g of protein) at some other point during the day.

CREATINE This amino acid helps increase adenosine triphosphate (ATP) and cell volume. Many people who take creatine notice that their muscles become engorged and that they feel stronger. Over the long term, creatine allows you to train with heavier weights or more reps, providing additional muscle stimulation and encouraging muscle growth.

Recommendation: The most effective time to take creatine is immediately following training. It should be combined with 50 g of whey protein and 50 g of simple carbs (such as dextrose/glucose). Taken in this manner, the amount of creatine needed per day is believed to be about 5 g for a 200-pound bodybuilder. Other sources might recommend

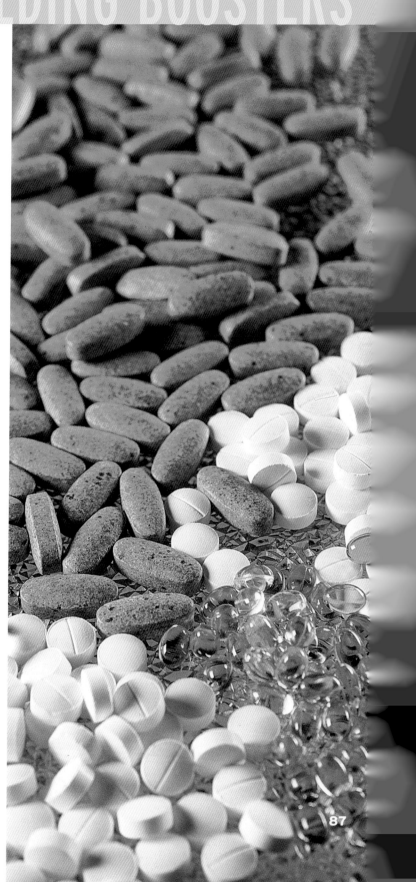

much larger dosages or "loading." But loading isn't necessary to experience the benefits of creatine.

GLUTAMINE The most prevalent free amino acid in muscle, glutamine is necessary for many vital physiological functions, including digestion, recovery and enhancing immune function. Weight training and other forms of exercise can deplete glutamine, forcing your body to pull amino acids from muscle tissue. Supplementing with glutamine provides your body with aminos it needs for recovery without depleting its stores. The overall effects are to spare muscle tissue and allow you to build even more.

   Recommendation: Glutamine can be taken throughout the day. We recommend consuming it first thing in the morning, between meals, after training and before bed. The average dosage at each of these times should be about 5 g. Overall, you should take 15-25 g per day. Many meal replacement powders and protein drinks have small amounts of glutamine added to them.

VITAMINS Everyone knows about vitamins, but few people know what they really are—small chemical structures that a body uses as nutrients. A deficiency in any of these may seriously impact both your bodybuilding training and your results. A diet rich in vegetables and fruits should cover most vitamin needs, but supplementing with the following vita-mins, either individually or in multipack form, will help ensure against deficiencies.

   Recommendation: Although there are convenient all-in-one multivitamins (and multiminerals), *FLEX* recommends vitamin packs or buying separate vitamins. By supplement-ing with each vitamin and mineral individually, you can be sure you're taking as much of each nutrient as you want or need. Basic recommendations are vitamin E, 400 to 800 international units (IU); vitamin C, 500-3,000 milligrams (mg), taken at no more than 1,000 mg at a time; B vitamins, 25-50 mg, taken with 400 micrograms (mcg) of folic acid; and vitamin A (beta carotene), 5,000 to 10,000 IU. Vitamins should be taken with solid-food meals when possible.

MINERALS Just as vitamins are micronutrients, so are minerals. Bodybuilders might be particularly susceptible to deficiencies in them brought on by the rigors of training.

The more active you are, the bigger you are, the more you sweat, the more calories you consume or the more you cut calories while dieting, the more minerals you need.

Recommendation: Different minerals might best be taken at different times. As with vitamins, we recommend a multipack containing the following minerals (or purchase them separately). The minerals and daily dosages recommended are calcium, 1 g; iron, 8 mg; iodine, 150 mcg; magnesium, 400 mg; zinc, 10-15 mg; and selenium, 100-400 mcg. As with vitamins, it's generally best to take minerals with solid-food meals.

SPECIALTY SUPPLEMENTS

Supplements can be excellent aids in helping you reach your goals. With that in mind, we've listed a few supplements that might help you address specific needs. These specialty items are the best way to complement your basic supplementation.

ESSENTIAL FATTY ACIDS Linolenic (omega-3) and linoleic (omega-6) fatty acids are essential fatty acids (EFAs). "Essential" means that your body cannot manufacture them from other fats, so you must get them through your diet. EFAs are crucial for increasing insulin sensitivity and insulin

We recommend a multipack containing the following minerals: calcium, iron, iodine, magnesium, zinc and selenium.

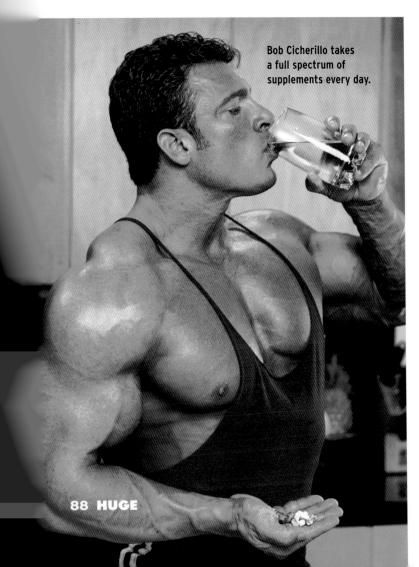

Bob Cicherillo takes a full spectrum of supplements every day.

binding to receptors in skeletal muscle, increased binding of growth factor (IGF-1) to skeletal muscle, decreasing cholesterol and triglyceride levels, moderating the release of cortisol, stimulating the release of growth hormone, promoting fat mobilization, and inhibiting bodyfat synthesis and storage.

Benefits: Good health and dietary support during low-carb dieting.

Recommendation: Eat fatty fish, such as salmon, sardines, mackerel and herring, two or three times a week. Also, work up to a tablespoon of flaxseed oil per one hundred pounds of bodyweight each day. If you prefer not to eat fish, you can supplement with fish oil (3-4 g per day). For easier digestion, take EFAs with your largest food meals of the day.

FIBER This indigestible carbohydrate (with zero calories) helps aid digestion. It increases the bulk of food, making it easier to digest dense foods, such as meat. It also helps your body derive more nutrients from the same quantity of food. Technically, fiber isn't a supplement (and neither is protein), but the way many bodybuilders add it to their nutritional regimens is akin to supplementation. Trainers should strive to get as much fiber as possible from sources such as oatmeal, whole grain bread, fruits and vegetables. But many athletes need more than that, and supplementing with it may be the best solution.

Benefit: Digestive support.

Recommendation: The more protein and the more calories you're eating, the more fiber you need. Using an over-the-

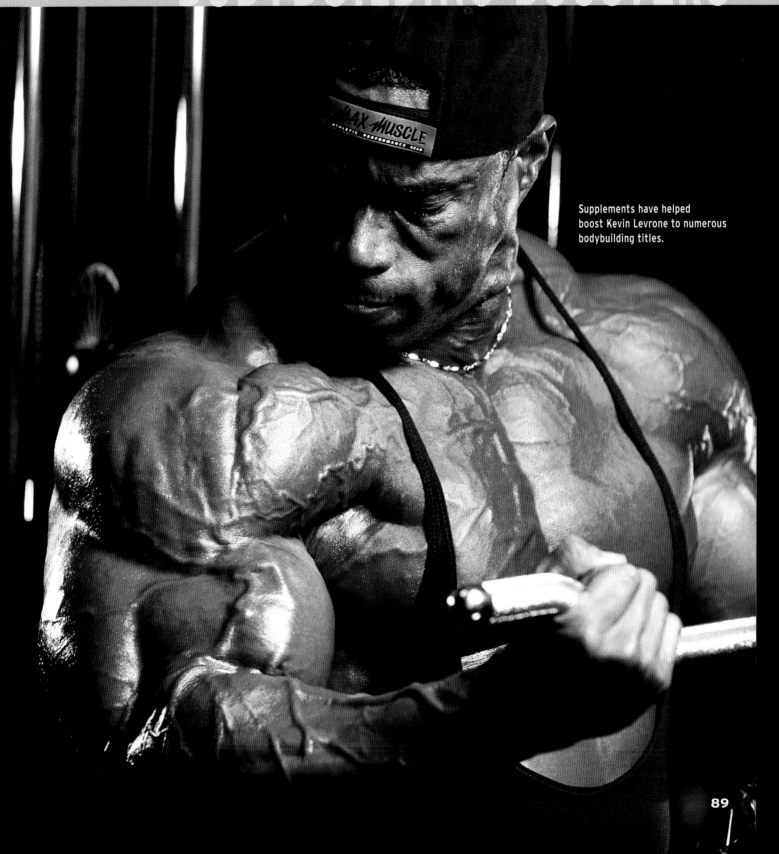

Supplements have helped boost Kevin Levrone to numerous bodybuilding titles.

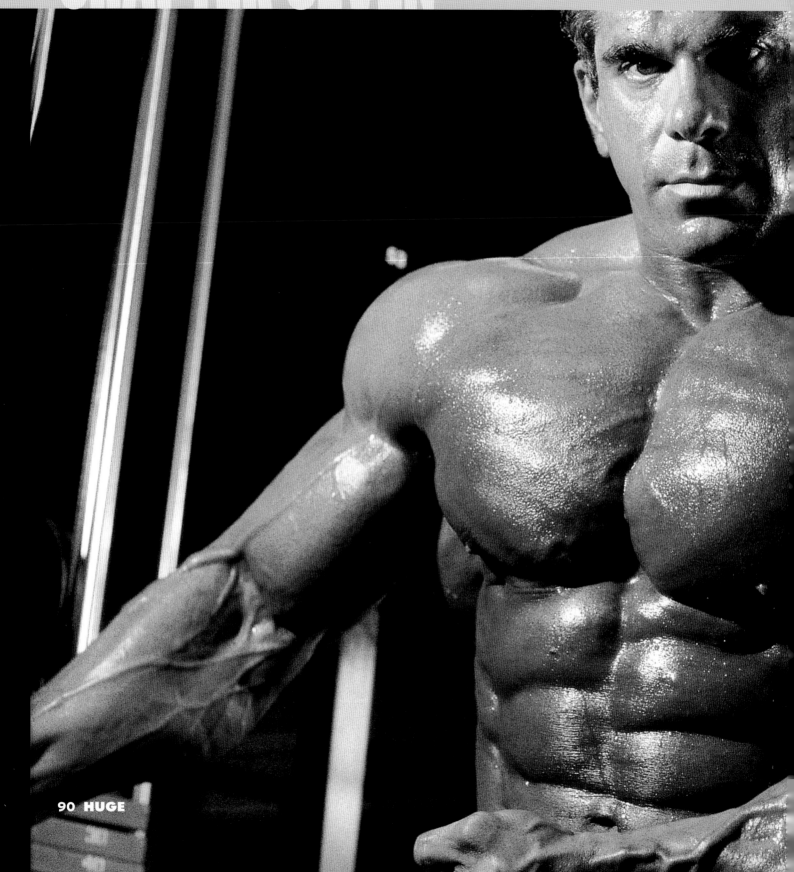

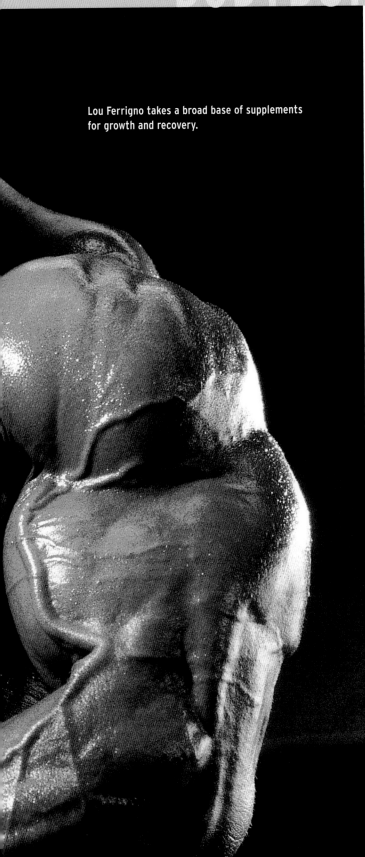

Lou Ferrigno takes a broad base of supplements for growth and recovery.

counter fiber supplement (such as Metamucil) twice a day may help improve digestion and digestive efficiency. Make certain to follow label recommendations for preparations. Fiber supplements should generally be well mixed in water. Additionally, bodybuilders should drink 12 to 16 ounces of water along with fiber drinks to provide the necessary solubility. You need at least 25 g a day — every day — of soluble and insoluble fiber from foods and supplements. Work up to that level gradually.

GLUCOSAMINE AND CHONDROITIN No matter how proper your form, heavy training eventually will take its toll on your joints and connective tissues. Glucosamine and chondroitin are components of connective tissue, particularly the cartilage inside joints. These supplements can help prevent and repair joint and connective-tissue damage. They are beneficial whether you already suffer joint pain or are seeking to prevent it.

Benefit: Joint support.

Recommendation: Often, these two are found in the same supplement. Some people prefer to take them separately; in that case, *FLEX* recommends 1,500 mg per day of glucosamine sulfate (or glucosamine hydrochloride) in three 500 mg dosages and 800-1,200 mg per day of chondroitin divided into two doses.

ZMA This supplement is a combination of zinc, magnesium aspartate and vitamin B in a proprietary blend. Clinical research using trained athletes as subjects strongly supports the theory that this combination can be effective in helping promote recovery for bodybuilders. Studies have demonstrated the effectiveness of ZMA in increasing anabolic hormone levels, including free testosterone and IGF-1, which might otherwise be suppressed in hard-training athletes. ZMA also improves sleep quality.

Benefit: Recovery.

Recommendation: Ideally, ZMA should be taken on an empty stomach shortly before bedtime to maximize its absorption and utilization, as well as to promote sleep. If your stomach is not empty at that time, take ZMA 20 to 30 minutes before your last meal or protein drink of the day. You'll get better results this way than if you take it with protein drinks. The dosage for the proprietary product is 30 mg zinc, 450 mg magnesium and 10.5 mg vitamin B_6.

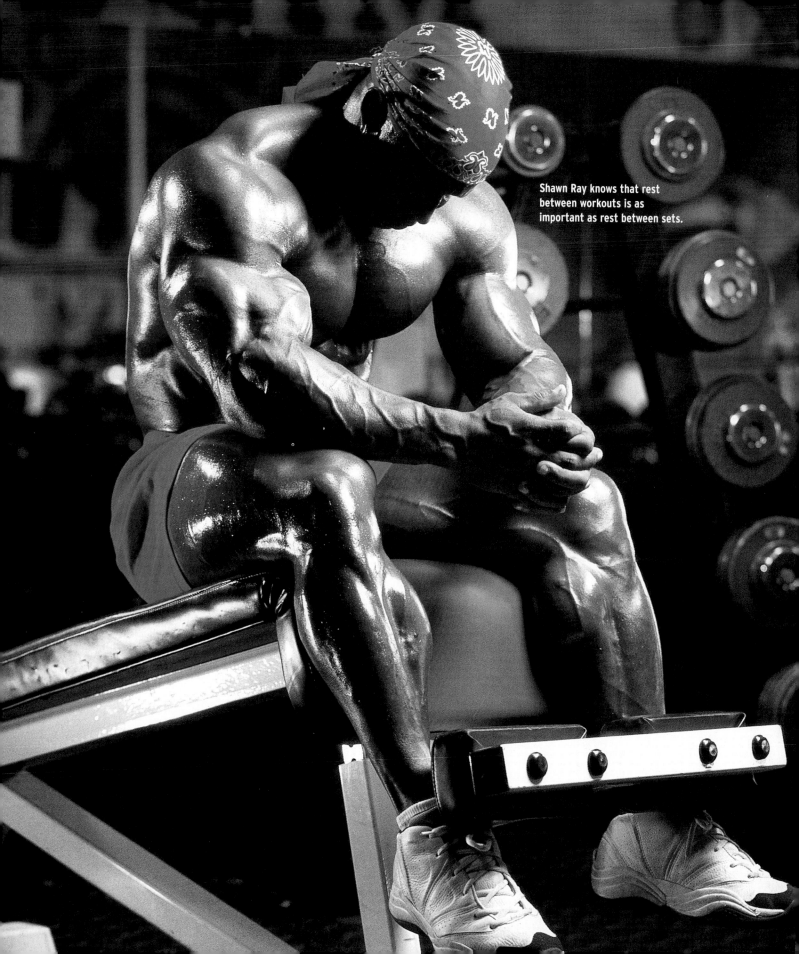

Shawn Ray knows that rest between workouts is as important as rest between sets.

Rest ASSURED

The importance of recuperation in your quest for mass

Bodybuilders follow training and nutrition advice to the letter, believing that if they eat all the right foods at the right times and successfully complete each exercise, set and rep, they will get huge. This is commendable, but all too often they overlook bodybuilding's crucial component: recuperation. The bottom line is you will not build optimum muscle if you do not allow your body the proper environment and amount of time to recover.

Recuperation is much more important and complex than most bodybuilders acknowledge.

The entire muscle-building process can be broken down into three phases: stimulation, recuperation and growth. Stimulation is achieved by putting a training stress on the body. After that stress is applied, the body begins the recuperation phase to recover from the workout. Only after the recuperation phase is complete does growth in muscle size (and strength) occur, and only after that phase is complete should the muscle be worked again. The most common mistake in bodybuilding is going back into the gym and working a muscle before it has completed the three phases of the muscle-building process.

Your bodybuilding endeavors can be broken down into three broad categories: workouts, nutrition and activities outside the gym. In assessing whether you are shortchanging yourself in a recuperation sense, apply the following recuperative strategies to each category.

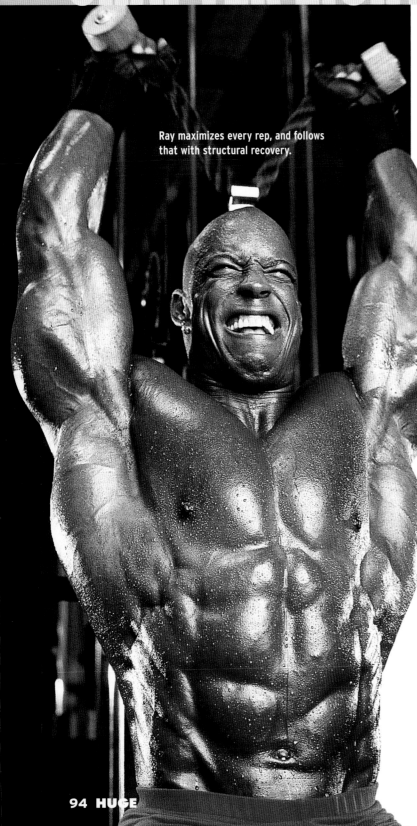

Ray maximizes every rep, and follows that with structural recovery.

WORKOUTS

LIMIT WEIGHT TRAINING TO FOUR DAYS A WEEK

The program in this book revolves around a four-day-a-week training schedule, which is an ideal frequency. It's easy to get caught up in the idea that training leads to growth; therefore, more training must lead to more growth. If you took that concept to its extreme, you would end up training every day. However, you would soon face burnout, because your body would not be getting sufficient recuperation time. This lack of recuperation not only applies to individual muscle groups, but also to the body's whole physiological system. As Dorian Yates put it, "The forgotten factor is that, for optimum recovery, the body's overall physiological and nervous system needs whole days at a time free from gym exertions to grow."

Physiologically, training causes stress to the muscles, which sets in motion recovery processes that operate after training. These processes take time and if you train too frequently, you derail your recuperation, bombarding your muscle tissues and physiological processes with more stress than they can handle (see "Red Flagging" at the end of this chapter for signs of overtraining).

Training four days a week is ideal. It allows your body three days a week for recuperation. Instead of training your body past the point where it can effectively respond with growth, put the time saved toward the rest strategies mentioned in this article.

LIMIT THE NUMBER OF EXERCISES PER WORKOUT

Not overtraining during individual sessions is key to maximizing muscle response. Since different exercises stimulate muscles differently, some eager amateurs strive to work a muscle in every possible way during each training session. The result? A catabolic response that tears down muscle tissue rather than builds it.

The exercise selection within this program is planned to give optimum stimulus to each muscle group. For large muscle groups such as chest and back, we prescribe three exercises; for small muscle groups such as biceps and triceps, we suggest two.

LIMIT THE NUMBER OF SETS PER WORKOUT

Maximal stimulation comes from the intensity you achieve during individual sets, not from the cumulative exhaustive effect of numerous sets. Remember, bodybuilding is an anaerobic sport, not an endurance one. The program in this book calls for 15 sets maximum per session for large bodyparts and fewer for small bodyparts. When you perform 20 or more sets for a bodypart, you are teaching your muscles to endure longer training sessions. A common byproduct of marathon training sessions is mentally pacing yourself and conserving energy during individual sets, which is the

nutrition to promote a full and fast recovery. Simple carbs help replenish glycogen stores in muscles that have been depleted by weight training, and protein provides amino acids to help repair structural damage that occurs in the muscles during weight training.

Within an hour of your postworkout intake of carbs and

You will not build optimum muscle if you do not allow your body the proper environment and amount of time to recover.

opposite of intensity. Pacing allows you to perform more sets and reps, but stimulates less muscle growth.

Instead, work with as much intensity as possible during fewer sets. This will stress your muscles more efficiently, and it will allow for more effective recuperation and growth. High-rep strategies should be avoided when you're going for growth. Using high reps can lead to increased definition, but it works against gaining muscular mass. Top-level body-builders use high-rep strategies when they are cutting up precontest, not while they are bulking up offseason.

NUTRITION

Nutrition is important not only for growth, but also for recuperation. Most bodybuilders are aware of the importance of eating for growth, but it's also worthwhile to understand how the following diet strategies impact recuperation.

POSTWORKOUT NUTRITION

Immediately after you train, you should consume 50-100 grams of simple carbs plus about 30-50 grams of protein. Your recovery from a workout begins right after you stop train-ing, and this is the ideal time to use

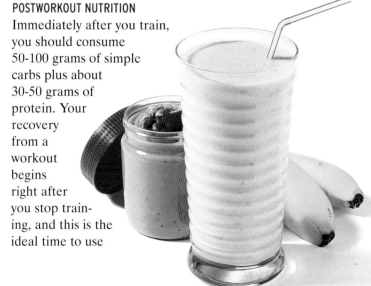

protein, you should have a full meal of protein, complex carbs and healthy fats. This second meal provides a steady stream of amino acids and other nutrients to keep the recuperation process in high gear. Feeding your body exactly what it needs at the right time is one of the most important steps in pro-moting recuperation.

EAT PLENTY OF PROTEIN

One of the most obvious bodybuilding tenets for growth is also key to recuperation. Each day, you need to supply your body with all the protein it needs for recovery: A daily intake of 1 to 1.5 grams of protein per pound of bodyweight split over five or six meals should be your goal. Loading up on quality postworkout nutrition is essential, but you also must follow through during the rest of the day. Before you go to bed, take in a small meal high in protein, but low in carbs. This can take the form of a protein drink or solid food, such as all-natural peanut butter, lean deli meat or a couple of soft-boiled eggs. Late-night protein intake provides your body with a stream of amino acids to assist the recuperative process.

EAT PLENTY OF COMPLEX CARBS

Carbohydrates help your muscles recover. After training, sugar or simple carbs start the process. Complex carbs give you a slower-burning form of energy to continue the process. Complex carbs consumed early in the morning also provide your body with a quality energy source for all your daily needs. Excellent sources of complex carbohydrates include brown rice, sweet potatoes and oatmeal.

EAT HEALTHY FATS

Moderate fat intake is important for a healthy body and for aiding recovery. Every cell membrane in the body is composed of fat. These membranes control the influx and

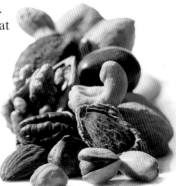

outflow of nutrients and waste. Providing your body with the fat it needs helps maintain cell integrity. In addition, dietary fats are crucial for immune function, hormone synthesis and a sense of well-being. A healthy bodybuilding diet contains sufficient mono- and polyunsaturated fats. Excellent sources of these nutrients include all-natural peanut butter, olives, avocados, many types of fish, vegetable oils, flaxseed oil, and nuts and seeds.

ACTIVITIES OUTSIDE THE GYM

GET PLENTY OF SLEEP

It's hard to quantify how much sleep an individual needs, but most bodybuilders do not get enough. When you have a life full of work, family and friends, as well as training and meal preparation, sleep is often the first thing to get short shrift. After a day that includes a hard training session, the average bodybuilder needs at least eight hours of sleep. Many people are functional on less, and so they burn the candle at both ends, sleeping six hours a night through the week and then playing catch-up on the weekend. That may be a good strategy for accomplishing daily goals, but it's not the best environment for muscle growth. During sleep, the body's recovery processes accelerate and growth hormone is released. When you cut short your sleep, you disturb the physiological mechanisms that allow you to maximize muscle potential.

Napping can be a time-efficient way to increase the amount of rest you get. Many people find that a short afternoon nap (30 minutes) provides them with even more energy than if they had slept an hour or two longer during the night. Of course, not many people have the luxury of taking afternoon naps, which makes nighttime slumber all the more important.

SCHEDULE PASSIVE RELAXATION

Ever wonder why your parents or grandparents spend most evenings sitting at home? As people age, downtime, particularly in the afternoon or evening, becomes more important. Similarly, people in their teens, 20s and 30s can benefit from relaxation. The goal isn't to turn yourself into a vegetable, but to recognize how much better you feel if you

SUPPLEMENTS FOR RECUPERATION

The following supplements are the most important in aiding your body in the recuperation process.

GLUTAMINE Glutamine is the bodybuilding supplement FLEX most highly recommends, primarily for its recuperative effects. Glutamine is the most prevalent amino acid in the body and, as such, is recruited for a wide array of physiological functions. When the body needs glutamine, it removes it from storage in muscle tissue or takes it from free-floating glutamine in your body. Supplementing with it helps keep your muscles intact by giving your body a readily available source.

Glutamine not only aids directly in recovery from training, but also enhances immune function and digestion. The impact the last two factors have on recovery can be tremendous and improving their function enhances bodybuilding gains.

CREATINE Most people use creatine because it engorges muscle tissue and may make them feel stronger. It also provides benefits for 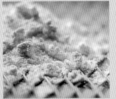 recovery. After training, creatine flows into the muscle tissue with water and nutrients. Creatine helps keep muscles full and ensures that the nutrients you have put into your body are delivered to your muscles.

Take creatine with a postworkout shake. If it's more convenient, you can take it on an empty stomach before training.

MULTIVITAMIN/MULTIMINERAL Vitamins and minerals are essential for physiological functions. A proper bodybuilding diet should provide all the vitamins and minerals a bodybuilder needs, but taking a multi can ensure that you have no deficits.

The antioxidant vitamins C and E help destroy free radicals released 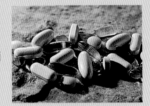 during training and help repair oxidative tissue damage caused by exercise. Minerals are essential for many bodily functions, and bodybuilders need higher doses of them because of the demands of training.

ZMA ZMA is a trademarked compound containing zinc and magnesium, two minerals that are particularly effective in helping the body recuperate. Taken on an empty stomach before bedtime, ZMA can help promote better sleep in addition to its recuperative powers.

spend an hour a day sitting quietly, enjoying a simple activity such as watching TV or reading.

Many pro bodybuilders have a reputation for being couch potatoes, but there's a good reason for that: The dividends of

help prime them for further activity. Professional athletes increasingly rely on these techniques to prevent and/or recover from injury. Older bodybuilders, with the benefit of hindsight, often say they wish they had taken better care of their

Your recovery from a workout begins right after you stop training, and this is the ideal time to use nutrition to promote a full and fast recovery.

relaxation are both immediate and long-term. In the short run, you may find you are able to sleep better at night by allowing your body to slow down as the day comes to an end. In the long run, you may notice you are less prone to injury and that you get a better response from your training.

SCHEDULE ACTIVE RELAXATION

Many forms of active relaxation can be enjoyable and recuperative. These include massage, acupuncture, yoga, stretching, steam baths or saunas, among others. Young bodybuilders don't put much time or effort into the longevity of their bodybuilding careers, but many pros do. Once you reach a certain age, often as young as your early 20s, you may notice that your body doesn't recuperate from training as quickly as it used to. Turning to active relaxation and recuperative strategies can help rejuvenate your body more quickly.

These techniques are not new-age hocus-pocus. They create physiological responses in the body and in the muscles that

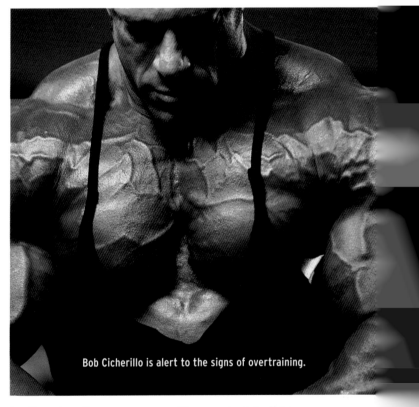

Bob Cicherillo is alert to the signs of overtraining.

RED FLAGGING

The following are the most common symptoms of overtraining.

- General lethargy and tiredness
- Sleeping fitfully or a disturbance in normal sleep patterns
- Irritability
- Loss of appetite
- Decreased strength levels
- Running out of steam before the end of a workout
- Dreading the next workout
- Joint aches

If you've noticed one or more of the above symptoms, you're probably overtraining. Stay out of the gym for 10 to 14 days, reassess your training and return to the gym with a program that factors in recuperation.

bodies when they were young. Younger bodybuilders can profit from the experience of older bodybuilders, using active relaxation techniques to promote healthier joints and muscles and to prolong their careers.

THE REST IS UP TO YOU

Recuperation is a key element in achieving optimum muscle growth. By adhering to the preceding guidelines, you will be ensuring that you are factoring in all the recuperation components necessary to facilitate your bodybuilding endeavors and your program will have taken a giant step forward.

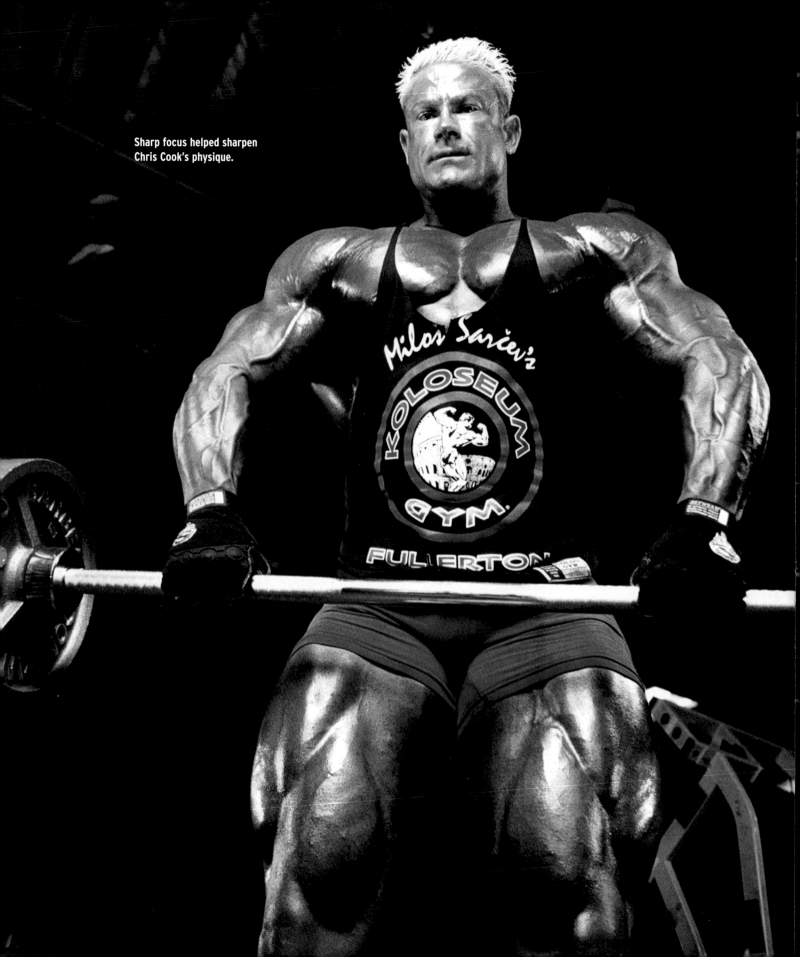

Sharp focus helped sharpen
Chris Cook's physique.

FOCUS

A motivational guide to keep your workouts fresh and challenging

By now you've realized that training takes a focused mindset. From following the Mass Attack program in Chapter 3, you will have already begun to get stronger and, at first, these increases in strength can be motivating in and of themselves. However, as your rate of strength gain begins to decrease or level off, you may find that your motivation also begins to wane a bit. You may find that your focus in the gym isn't always what it should be as this phase of the program begins to test the boundaries of your strength and mental resolve.

This chapter is devoted to providing methods for you to maintain optimum focus during a heavy lifting phase. Staying motivated is key to enabling you to make the greatest gains in strength and, ultimately, muscle. These are the guidelines that the pros have identified as being the most helpful.

KEEP A TRAINING LOG

Daily examination of a training journal can be among the most motivational of all bodybuilding tools. If you aren't already recording your workouts, begin doing so now. Of particular importance is writing down all the sets, reps, exercises and poundages you use. Training logs are crucial for giving you a frame of reference and for allowing you to look back to see the progress you've made. Such reviews hep you to understand that progress does not take the form of one consistent upward curve, but rather a series of peaks and plateaus. If you find yourself at a sticking point, reviewing your training journal can motivate you by reinforcing the fact that sticking points are eventually conquered.

2 DEVELOP A PREPARATION RITUAL

As with anything in life, how you prepare affects how you perform. Bodybuilders who establish rituals to help them prepare for their workouts find that they are much more focused during their training sessions.

Six-time Mr. Olympia Dorian Yates is a strong advocate of preparation rituals. "A few hours before my workout, I review my diary and target the sets, reps and poundages I will use that day. I visualize myself doing the exercises. I see the plates on the bar and imagine how heavy the weight's going to feel. I see the bar

Staying motivated is key to enabling you to make the greatest gains.

bend, and I envision how hard I'll have to push to move it. By the time I enter the gym, it's like I just have to insert a prerecorded tape and rubber-stamp the workout. This preamble is to ensure that I'm 100% focused on the job at hand and won't arrive at the gym with the attitude of 'OK, what shall I do today?' "

Individual rituals can vary tremendously. Yours may involve aspects of nutrition, supplementation, meditation, forms of warm-ups or any other activity or environmental shift that encourages you to focus on your workout and bring all the intensity you can muster to your training.

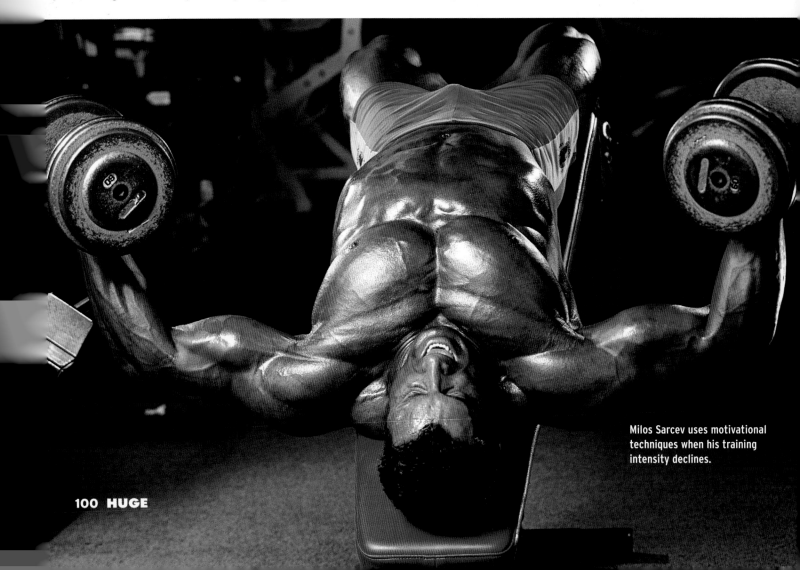

Milos Sarcev uses motivational techniques when his training intensity declines.

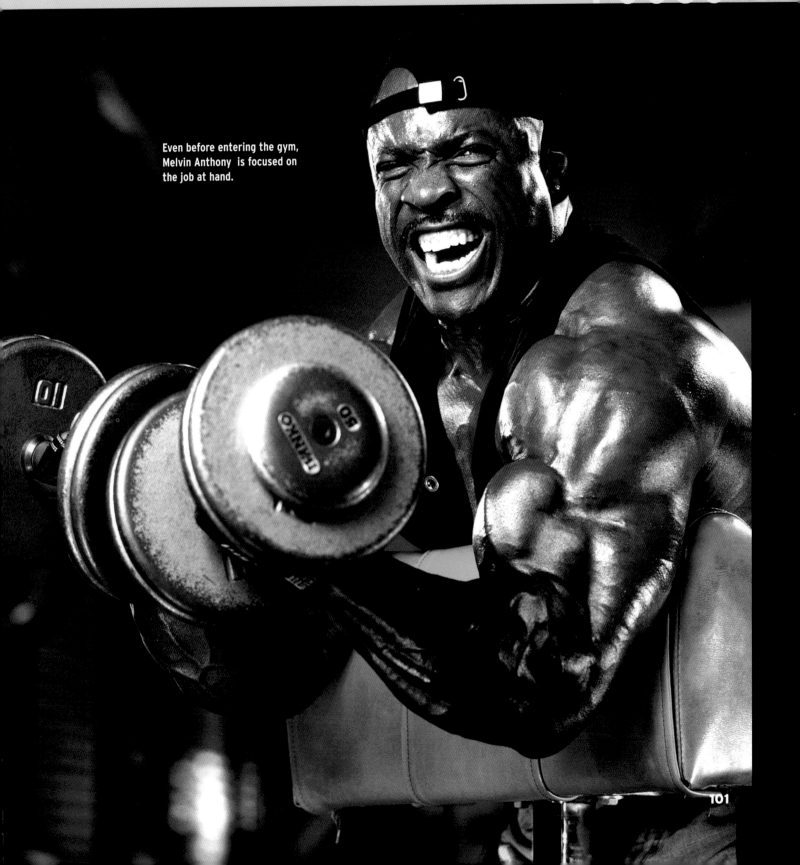

Even before entering the gym, Melvin Anthony is focused on the job at hand.

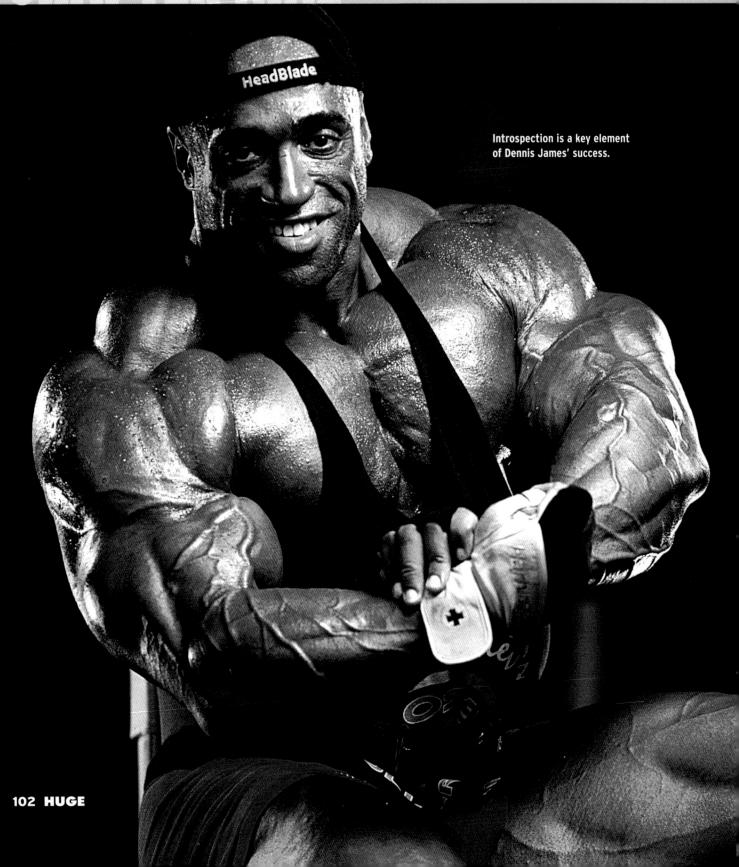

Introspection is a key element of Dennis James' success.

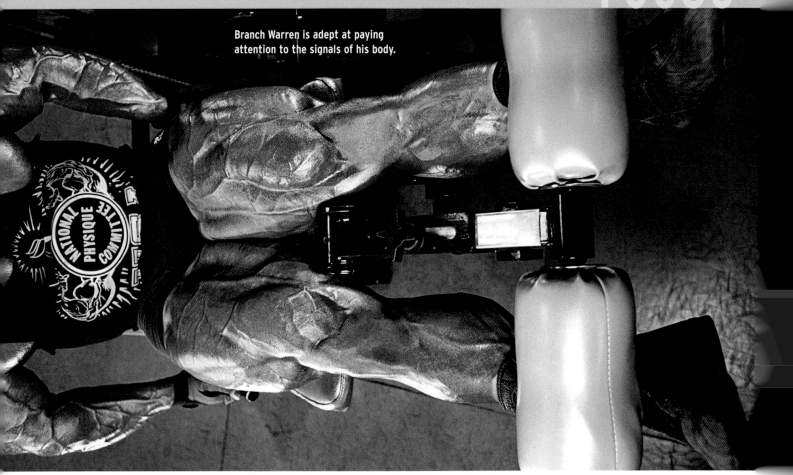

Branch Warren is adept at paying attention to the signals of his body.

3 DON'T BLINDLY FOLLOW YOUR TRAINING PROTOCOL

The purpose of your workout is to serve your body, not for your body to serve the workout. Many bodybuilders become impeded by blindly trying to follow a preset routine rather than focusing on the larger goal of improving their physiques. When you become a slave to individual workouts, you have lost sight of your true goals.

Part of the preparation ritual is to ascertain what your training protocol should be for that day. Dorian explains how he approaches this concept. "Before each workout, I'll ask myself things like 'Do I feel strong today, or am I a little tired?' I'll also assess whether I have fully recuperated from the previous work-out, and I might make the decision not to train that day. Other times, I'll actually be warming up in the gym before realizing 'No, today's not my day. I'm not fresh enough to give 100%.' If that's the case, I'll leave the gym without a shred of guilt. I don't look upon my training as a discipline that I have to complete X amount of times a week. A workout is undertaken for the sole purpose of stimulating muscle growth, and if I'm not fully recuperated, I won't stimulate muscle growth. I know that if I take that day off, I can come back the next day totally motivated for having a tremendous workout."

4 STAY ATTUNED TO YOUR BODY

The human body constantly sends signals to the brain, and often we override those signals because they are not compatible with the goals we've set for ourselves. Becoming the best bodybuilder you can possibly be entails learning when to listen and obey these signals, and when to override them. Strive to err on the side of listening to your body over ignoring its messages. Nothing derails progress faster than injury or overtraining, and nothing causes these more readily than ignoring what your body tells you.

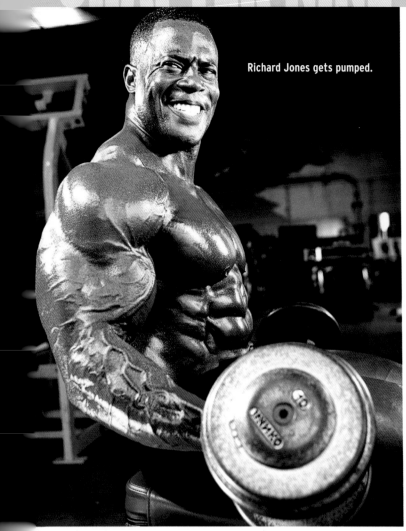

Richard Jones gets pumped.

your muscles; the aim is light training. These pump days will help keep you focused on your overall goal of increasing your strength so that when you move into the next training phase, you will be able to use your increased strength to help sculpt an even more impressive physique.

6 ADJUST YOUR DIET TO SUPPORT POWER TRAINING

Bodybuilding diets are notoriously difficult for the discipline they demand. The good news is that during the power phase, you do not need to rigorously adhere to the precepts of a strict bodybuilding diet. The purpose of the workout in Chapter 10 is to increase strength, so you need to adjust your diet to support that goal.

Although you do not want to add excessive bodyfat, you do want to provide your body with all the nutrients it needs for growth and recovery. *FLEX* continues to stress the importance of a diet high in protein for muscle building and complex carbs for sustained energy. However, while you're in a strength-building phase, you may want to include more fat in your diet. *FLEX* recommends taking in approximately 15% of your daily calories in the form of healthy fats while on a pure bodybuilding diet. While you're in a strength-building phase, increase your fat consumption to 20-25%. This can be attained by including more red meat in place of skinless chicken breast and whole eggs instead of egg whites. However, don't go overboard—try to stick with unsaturated fats.

Consuming more fat during a power-training program provides you with many benefits. Fats help make you strong by providing your body with the necessary components to create an ideal hormonal environment for increasing strength and promoting recovery. Also, fats provide your body with a sense of well-being and satiety. In short, they make you happier, and a happy bodybuilder is a motivated bodybuilder.

Conversely, take advantage of days when you feel your best. Push yourself to achieve or exceed preset goals, but do so in the context of the workout.

5 USE PUMP WORKOUT DAYS TO STAY MOTIVATED

As you transition into the three-month power program in Chapter 10, pump workout days will help serve as a motivational tool as they provide an improvisational relief from the rigorous mental and physical challenge of your power-day workouts. Make pump days fun so that they provide training variety as a precursor to launching into the next power-workout day.

To that end, you should think of your pump days as active rest. The aim is not to take your sets to failure and fatigue

7 EAT FOR INDIVIDUAL TRAINING SESSIONS

Your body needs more fuel (and motivation) for power-training days than it does for the other days of the week. Adjust your diet to give your body what it needs. Try consuming a large breakfast of ham and eggs on your hardest workout days and see if you don't notice an increased motivation to train then. In addition, eat 100-200 grams of complex carbs from a source such as oatmeal. Complex carbs will help provide your

Make pump days fun so that they provide training variety as a precursor to launching into the next power-workout day.

body with a steady release of slow-burning energy throughout the day. Even if you don't train until evening, a fully satisfying breakfast followed by a sizable lunch of roasted chicken or red meat and more complex carbs will fuel your workout more effectively than a standard bodybuilding diet designed to help reduce bodyfat.

8 USE ERGOGENIC AIDS ONLY AS AN OCCASIONAL BOOST

Many bodybuilders use ergogenic aids, such as ephedrine and caffeine, to enhance their workouts or to encourage fat loss. These supplements are potentially quite motivating; however, many bodybuilders use them in a manner that provides very little boost. When you take an ergogenic aid consistently before each workout, your body comes to rely upon that external boost as part of an ordinary workout, much like a person who drinks three cups of coffee every morning simply to wake up.

A far better strategy is to use ergogenics sparingly before your most difficult workouts. Instead of using them every time you train, try taking them only once a week—for your squat day one week, then for your bench-press power day the next. A moderate dosage taken intermittently will have a more dramatic impact on your workouts than consistent regular use of ergogenics.

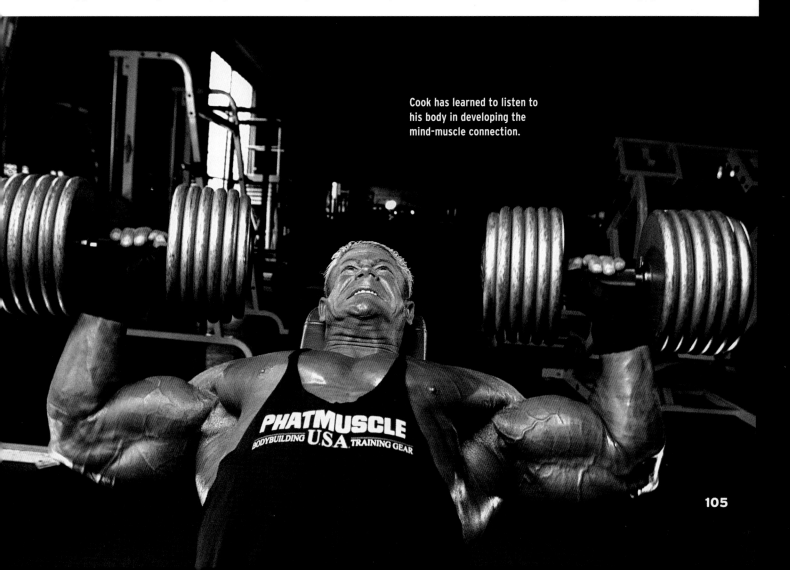

Cook has learned to listen to his body in developing the mind-muscle connection.

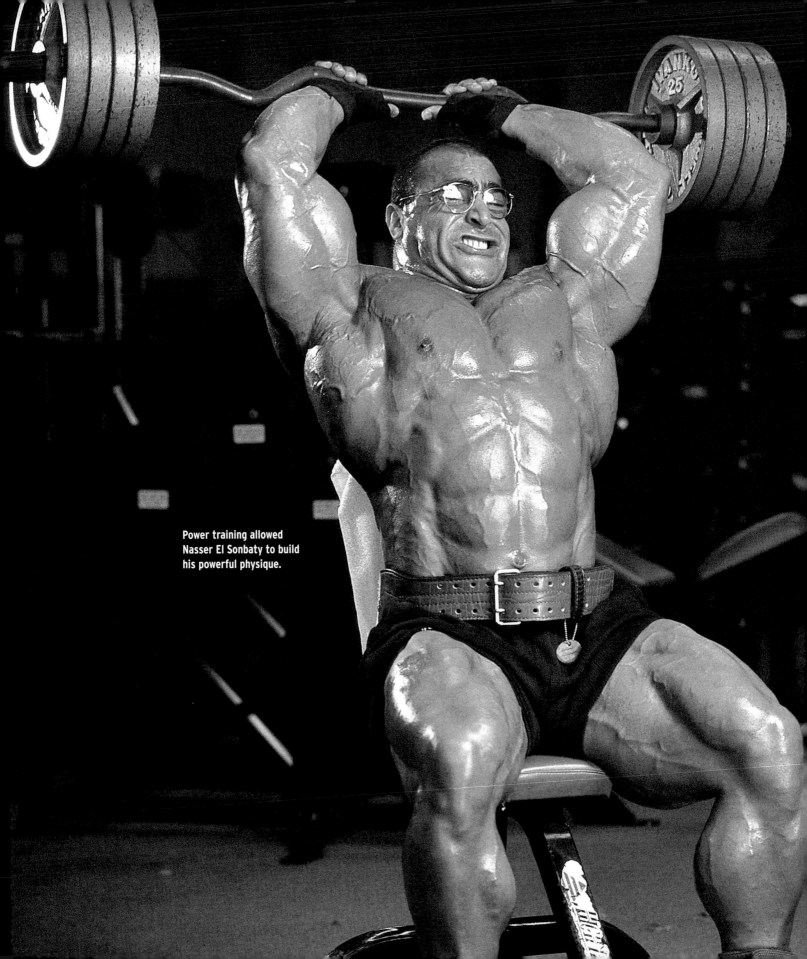

Power training allowed
Nasser El Sonbaty to build
his powerful physique.

Three-Month POWER PROGRAM

Pack on muscle size and increase strength with this 13-week Power Surge

The 13-week training program in Chapter 3 emphasized using perfect form while developing a mental connection with the muscle being worked. We also stressed rest periods of only a minute or so between sets. The overall thrust of the 13-week segment was to introduce you to the mindset of internalizing the bodybuilding process, so that instead of concentrating on the weight being lifted, you focused on the muscles moving the weight.

Now it's time to take it up a notch. You've laid the foundation and you're ready for liftoff into an intense power trip: a new 13-week program, based on lifts and periodization methods used by powerlifters.

Despite the fact that *FLEX* regularly says bodybuilding is not powerlifting, we can learn a lot from the beefy strongmen who partake of it. Powerlifters are dedicated athletes who have brought a science to lifting ever-escalating poundages and — listen up — know a thing or two about getting big. They don't give a flying dumbbell about V-taper waistlines, and people might not beg them to take their shirts off to pose, but their priority is not physique, it's totals! For the next 13 weeks, that will be your priority, too.

The weighty worlds of bodybuilding and powerlifting once

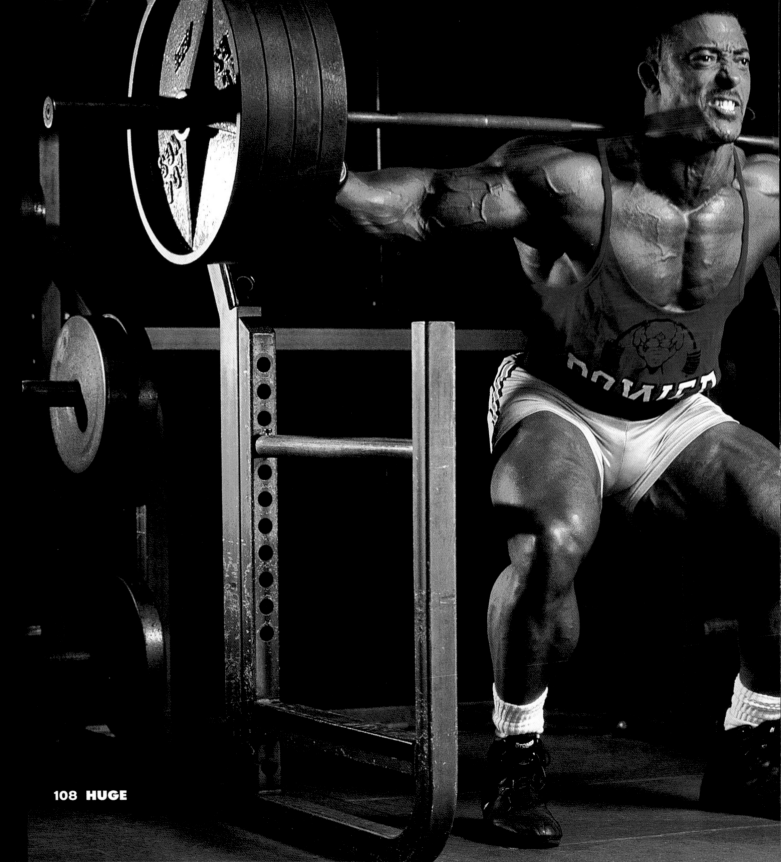

These are the days for building awesome size and power. Make that your focus.

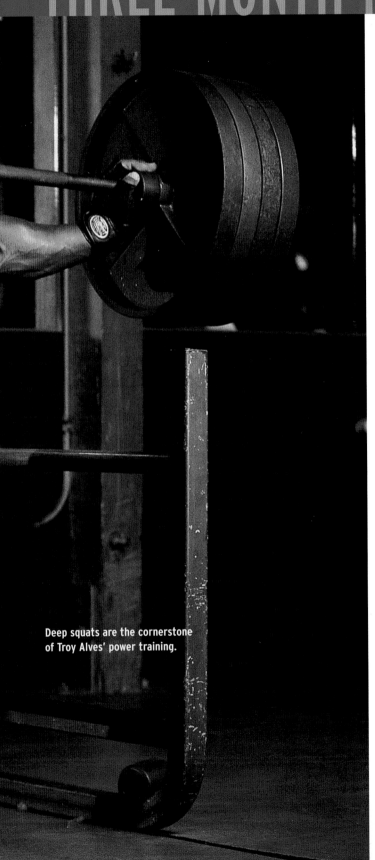

Deep squats are the cornerstone of Troy Alves' power training.

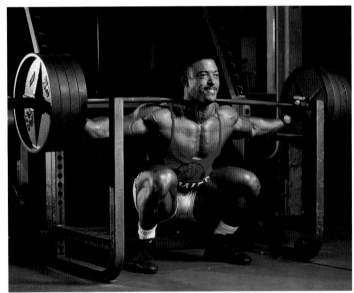

were closer. At one time, bodybuilders were as much into the numbers game as today's powerlifters. Physique contests in the '40s, '50s and '60s frequently included strength components — the two went hand in lifting glove. Sergio Oliva cut his teeth as an Olympic lifter, and other Mr. Olympias, such as Arnold Schwarzenegger, Franco Columbu and even Ronnie Coleman, competed as powerlifters. Now, it's rare to find power training in a physique program. In this era of specialized techniques and supplement gurus' magic potions, the basics of powerlifting have been left behind in bodybuilding training.

That's a shame, because adopting powerlifting techniques for bodybuilding will bring you closer to your physique goals than you've ever imagined possible. We're going to show you how.

GOING MENTAL

Bodybuilders can learn many things from powerlifters, the most important of which is mental attitude. When a power-lifter goes under a plate-loaded squat bar for a limit lift, his mental tenacity and will to succeed are as important as the strength of his muscles. He must first beat that weight mentally if he has any chance of getting his muscles to move the damn thing. Likewise, the success you reap from this 13-week Power Surge will ultimately depend on the level of mental tenacity you bring to your workouts. You must adopt the powerlifting attitude that you, not the weight, are the master, and that you will not fail in your lifts.

The Power Surge (see the charts on pages 125 and 126) utilizes a four-day-per-week lifting regimen, divided into "power" and "pump" days. You need three days off per week, doing absolutely nothing — no aerobics, no gymnastics, no Broadway performances — to recover from these mind-bending workouts.

Power days (Monday and Friday) are the hard workouts, in which you utilize basic compound exercises in the powerlifting tradition. The three powerlifting movements — squats, bench presses and deadlifts — form the core of the workouts. It is in these three lifts that you can move the most weight and shock your body into optimum strength and muscle growth. Therein lies the essence of the Power Surge: As you get stronger on these three lifts, you will get bigger!

On pump days (Tuesday and Thursday), you go into the gym with the goal of pumping the designated muscles with higher-rep sets, supersets or any means of getting a pump. Pump days allow you to flush your muscles with blood. This actively boosts recovery by nourishing your tissues. It feels good, too.

CONTROLLED POWER

If you're used to bodybuilding training — lifting to failure and waiting for that satisfying pump — fuggedaboutit. On power days, you're going to move heavy weight for low reps and take long rests between sets. You won't train to failure — you'll train to just short of failure, using maximum poundages to build strength throughout your physique by employing all muscles in the basic lifts. You'll do percentages of your one-rep maximum (1RM) while using very strict form. That's the central rule that applies in bodybuilding and powerlifting. Screwing with form during heavy powerlifting exercises can lead to severe injuries and a great deal of humiliation in the gym. Maintain perfect form!

Use the first week to experiment and discover your 1RM on all lifts in the program. It's not a perfect science, but do

your best during this time to determine how much to lift on hard days. Later in this feature, we provide guidelines for determining your 1RM.

Familiarize yourself with the basic movements, especially the three crucial powerlifting exercises: squats, deadlifts and

POWER EATING

Nobody ever got bigger by eating less. Note what your average daily caloric intake is before you begin the Power Surge and increase that amount by 5-10% (using nutritious foods). Ensure that your diet contains sufficient protein, which is the nutritional bedrock of building muscle. A recommended macronutrient profile would be 50% of calories from unrefined carbs (more emphasis on fruits and vegetables than on starches); 30% from protein sources; and 20% from fats. Strive for four to eight meals daily. Good supplement choices are protein powders and meal-replacement powders, creatine, glutamine, and a good multivitamin/multimineral pack.

bench presses. Follow the prescripts of this program strictly and build up slowly with these three lifts. Remember, on power days you're not training to failure or going for a pump. You're recruiting many different muscles to move the weight to improve strength. Stronger muscles mean bigger muscles.

Powerlifting is bread-and-butter stuff — a basic-training style that builds foundations for athletic success. Bodybuilding training should incorporate variety to keep things interesting; this power-and-pump program gives you that.

Now it's time to begin the ultimate Power Surge.

POWER POINTS: NINE STEPS TO THE ULTIMATE POWER SURGE

1. TRAINING FREQUENCY
- Train four times per week in a two-on, one-off, two-on, two-off rotation. This schedule maximizes efficiency, recovery and productivity.
- We have assigned the training days as Monday, Tuesday, Thursday and Friday, but you can use a different day split as long as you adhere to the rotation.
- Mondays and Fridays are your power days. Tuesdays and Thursdays are your pump days.
- Take three days of total rest during the week. On off-days, don't do any strenuous exercise, including cardio. Conserve your energy for the workout days.

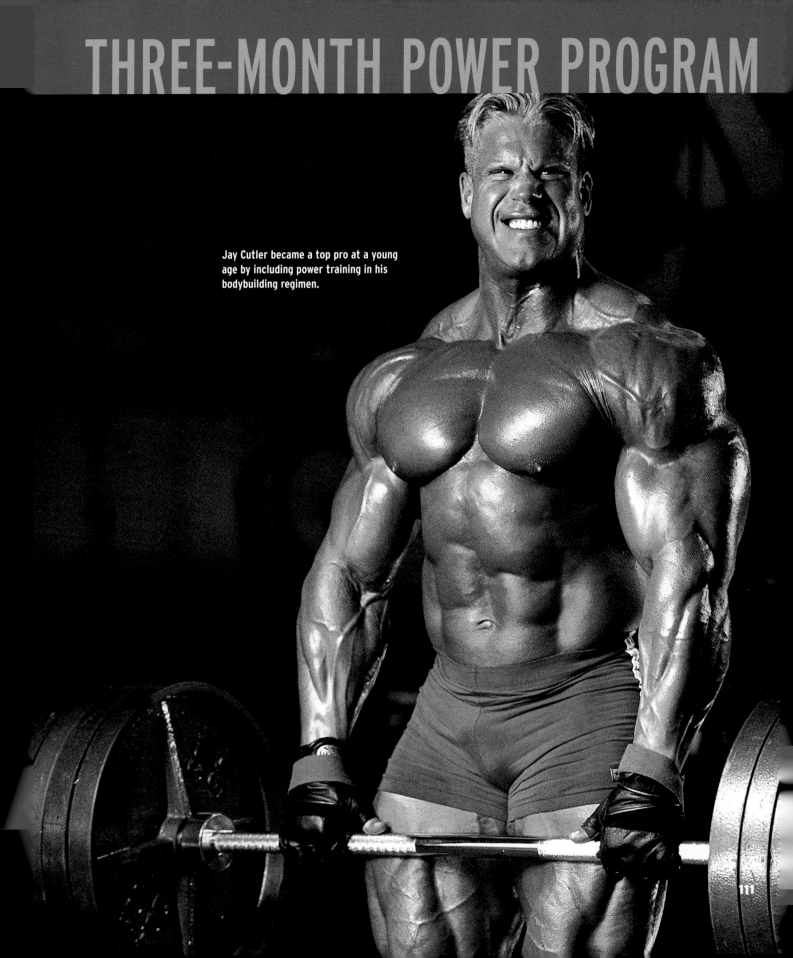

Jay Cutler became a top pro at a young age by including power training in his bodybuilding regimen.

By getting stronger on squats, deadlifts and bench presses during these 13 weeks, you will be getting bigger.

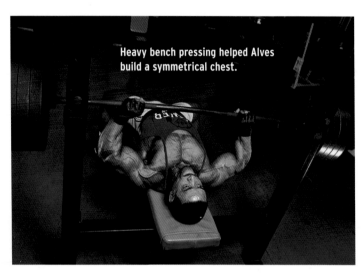

Heavy bench pressing helped Alves build a symmetrical chest.

2. BODYPART SPLIT

■ Train each bodypart twice per week (see "Power Surge: Chart One" for the sequence), once in power mode and once in pump mode.

■ The bodypart split is based on a push-pull format. Train the main pushing muscles (chest, shoulders and triceps) on Tuesdays and Fridays, and the other muscles on Mondays and Thursdays.

■ Do chest and shoulders in one workout so the delicate shoulder joint is put under direct pressing stress on only two days.

■ To ensure that chest and shoulders get equal treatment, alternate training those bodyparts first from workout to workout.

3. PRINCIPLES OF THE POWER WORKOUT

■ On Mondays and Fridays, train with power movements, the strength monsters that laid the foundation for the eye-popping size of Ronnie Coleman, Arnold Schwarzenegger and many of the other all-time great bodybuilders.

■ Squats, deadlifts and bench presses are the big three, the basic compound exercises that work ancillary

muscles and enable you to handle the most weight and, therefore, stimulate optimum strength and muscle size.

■ In this low-rep program, always use perfect form while going through a complete range of motion. End the set when you can no longer maintain perfect form, because that means you've lost the ability to move the weight by sheer muscle power alone.

■ Never go to failure on power days. These are the days for building awesome size and power. Make that your focus.

■ Get psyched for your power days! Remember, mental strength will determine your progress. Before going to the gym, get yourself into a mental zone, determined to hit your targets.

4. EXERCISE SELECTION

■ The power days emphasize the basic meat-and-potatoes strength builders: squats (for legs), deadlifts (for back) and flat barbell bench presses (for chest). These three powerlifting movements are the ultimate compound exercises for developing total-body strength and power. By getting stronger on squats, deadlifts and bench presses during these 13 weeks, you will be getting bigger.

■ Other power choices for max strength development include cable rows (for back), barbell or machine shrugs

POWER MATH

Since we require you to lift varying percentages of your one-rep max (1RM) in the Power Surge program, we thought we'd give you a hand in figuring it all out. The first step is figuring out your 1RM. Do that by finding your six-rep max, that is, the poundage with which you reach failure, using perfect form, after six reps. Once you've determined that weight, multiply it by 1.25. The resulting poundage will represent your 1RM. This formula (multiplying by 1.25) works no matter what poundage you top out at after six reps.

Next, base all the poundage percentages we prescribe on your 1RM. If you need to determine 60% of your 1RM, multiply your 1RM by .60; if you need to determine 85% of your 1RM, multiply your 1RM by .85. And do yourself a favor: Don't waste mental energy or paper trying to sort this all out — use a calculator!

(for traps), barbell curls (for biceps), standing calf raises (for calves), seated barbell presses (for shoulders) and lying triceps extensions (for triceps).

5. PREP FOR POWER

■ The goal during the power days of the first week is to experiment with poundages to determine your one-rep max (1RM) on each exercise. During this 1RM assessment week, start with light warm-up sets and progress to heavier weights. Use perfect form and a full range of motion.

■ Here is a guide to determine your 1RM: Identify the amount you can lift for six perfect reps (with a seventh being impossible) of each power-day exercise. That equates to roughly 80% of your 1RM. Therefore, if you squat 200 pounds for six reps max, multiply that poundage by 1.25, and the result, 250 pounds, would be a reasonable estimate of your 1RM. Use 1.25 as your multiplier no matter how much weight you lift for those six reps.

■ Since the goal of this program is to get stronger, your 1RM will gradually increase as the weeks tick by. Therefore, for bench presses, deadlifts and squats, you should reassess your 1RM after weeks four and eight, and adjust your poundages accordingly. This reassessment (determining your six-rep max) is best done at the beginning of a pump workout.

6. CYCLING THE POUNDAGES

■ This 13-week regimen does not follow the usual linear progression of poundages (see "Power Surge: Chart Two"). Instead, you'll use proven powerlifting methods.

■ Powerlifters have discovered that the optimum way to gain strength is by cycling poundages in a two-steps-forward, one-step-backward formula, rather than trying to maintain a consistently progressive lifting curve. That means oscillating from higher to lower percentages of your 1RM. For instance, in the fifth week, your top weight is at 85% of your max, but in the sixth, drop down to 70%.

■ This oscillation also occurs within specific workouts. For instance, in the fifth week, you'll handle heavy weights in the third and fourth sets (2x6 at 80% of max), then cut back in the sixth set (1x8 at 50% of max).

■ Note that for some bodyparts, you do not follow the

POWER SURGE: CHART ONE

BODYPART SPLIT, EXERCISE AND TRAINING-INTENSITY GUIDE

POWER DAYS

DAY*	BODYPART	EXERCISE	POWER THRESHOLD TO FOLLOW[†]
Monday	Legs	Squats	Weeks 1-13
	Back	Deadlifts	Weeks 1-13
		Cable rows	Weeks 1-8, and stay at that workload[††]
	Traps	Machine or barbell shrugs	Weeks 1-8, and stay at that workload
	Biceps	Barbell curls	Weeks 1-5, and stay at that workload**
	Calves	Standing calf raises	Weeks 1-8, and stay at that workload
Friday	Chest	Barbell bench presses	Weeks 1-13
	Shoulders	Seated barbell presses	Weeks 1-8, and stay at that workload
	Triceps	Lying triceps extensions	Weeks 1-5, and stay at that workload
	Abs	Leg raises	For maintenance, do 3 sets, 20 reps each

PUMP DAYS

DAY	BODYPART	RECOMMENDED EXERCISE
Tuesday	Shoulders	Dumbbell presses
		Lateral raises
	Chest	Incline dumbbell presses
		Flat-bench flyes
	Triceps	Cable pressdowns
	Abs	Crunches (for maintenance, do 3 sets, 20 reps each)
Thursday	Legs	Leg presses
		Lunges
	Back	Barbell rows
		Pulldowns
	Traps	Upright rows
	Biceps	Seated alternate curls
		Incline curls
	Calves	Seated calf raises

* *Rest completely on Sunday, Wednesday and Saturday.*
[†] *See Chart Two for a full guide to the sets, reps and percent of one-rep max you should aim for.*
[††] *For cable rows, shrugs, calf raises and seated barbell presses, once you achieve the threshold prescribed for the eighth week, stay at that workload for the remainder of the Power Surge.*
** *For biceps and triceps, once you reach the threshold noted for week five, stay at that workload for the remainder of the Power Surge.*
Note: In your Tuesday and Friday workouts, alternate chest and shoulders as the first bodypart you work.

POWER SURGE: CHART TWO

SET, REP AND POUNDAGE GUIDE FOR POWER DAYS

This chart shows the sets, reps and weight schemes to use, based on your one-rep max. These should be applied to all "power" movements, but not to your "pump" training. The core compound movements, including squats, deadlifts and bench presses, follow the full 13-week regimen. Other movements, such as cable rows, shrugs, calf raises and seated barbell presses, peak at week eight — once you reach that workload for those exercises, stay at that threshold of training for subsequent weeks. For triceps and biceps, you reach the power threshold at week five and, once you have reached that point, you should stay at that workload for the remainder of the program. After weeks four and eight, reevaluate your one-rep max and adjust your weights accordingly.

WEEK	SETS*	REPS	WEIGHT (ONE-REP MAX %)
1	Use this week to assess your one-rep max, as described in step 5, page 125		
2	3	10	65%
3	4	8	70%
4	1	6	80%
	2	8	70%
5	1	5	55%
	1	4	85%
	2	6	80%
	1	4	75%
	1	8	50%
6	3	5	70%
7	2	6	80%
	1	6	75%
8	3	4	85%
	1	4	80%
9	1	4	85%
	1	6	80%
	1	4	75%
10	1	3	55%
	2	3	90%
	1	4	85%
	1	3	75%
	1	8	50%
11	3	3	70%
12	1	2	90%
	1	2	80%
	1	2	75%
13	1	2	95%
	1	1	90%
	1	2	80%
	1	6	55%

* Warm-up sets are not represented in the power set and rep schemes shown here. Do at least two light warm-up sets of 20 reps before attempting your first power set. Don't perform so many reps that you fatigue or "pump" your muscles. Save that style of training for your pump-days training.

13-week progression. See the introductory paragraph in "Power Surge: Chart Two."

7. PRINCIPLES OF THE PUMP WORKOUT

■ On Tuesdays and Thursdays, let loose and enjoy the pure pleasure of pumping blood into your muscles. This is done by hitting each bodypart for about six sets of eight to 10 reps in one or two exercises of your choice.

■ Use poundages that equate to 65% of your 1RM.

■ In the pump mode, take short rests (90 seconds at most) between sets so that the pump is maximized.

■ Don't go higher than 10 reps on your sets. You still want to handle decent poundages that will stimulate muscle hardness and density.

■ Do supersets, giant sets or whatever format tickles your fancy.

■ Relax the rigid mental focus you attain for power days. Go into the gym with the objective of enjoying the sensation of making the blood engorge the targeted muscle groups.

■ In "Power Surge: Chart One," we've made some recommendations for specific exercises to use on pump days, but feel free to substitute your favorites.

8. REST PERIODS BETWEEN POWER AND PUMP SETS

■ Remember, for power days the focus is on moving the heaviest weights possible with perfect form within a prescribed rep scheme. It is not about getting a pump.

■ On power days, rest at least four minutes between sets, so your muscles fully recover from one set, letting you exert maximum power in the next.

■ When the going really gets heavy in week nine and on, rest longer between sets, if need be. On power days, you should rest up to 10 minutes between working main bodyparts.

■ The goal on pump days is to get a maximum pump, so, as we said before, rest 90 seconds or less between sets.

9. SAFETY FIRST!

■ On power days, when you're using extremely heavy weights in low-rep schemes, always have a spotter ready to step in and assist you. This is absolutely essential on squats, bench presses, shoulder presses and lying triceps extensions.

THREE-MONTH POWER PROGRAM

Long rests between power sets allow Milos Sarcev to use perfect form with the heaviest weight possible.

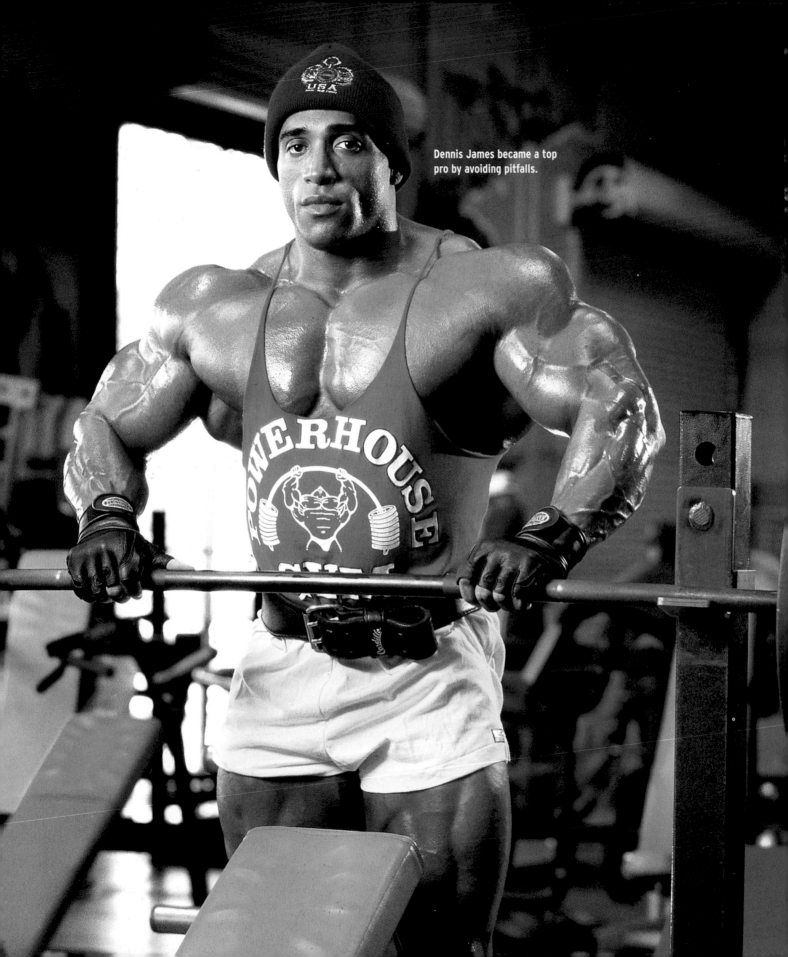

Dennis James became a top
pro by avoiding pitfalls.

Training HAZARDS

Here are seven pitfalls to watch out for in the gym, and how to avoid them

You might not be getting absolutely everything you can from your regimen.

The following checklist gives you a frame of reference for determining whether or not you're veering into one of these hazards at the gym. Use our detours to train around them.

HAZARD #1: OVERTRAINING
DETOUR: KEEP YOUR TRAINING MODERATE

When growth is your goal, it's easy to buy into the all-or-nothing training mentality. As we have pointed out, training too frequently, too long, or using too many sets, reps or exercises can all lead to overtraining. To get the most from your program, it's imperative that you stay within the

training parameters we've outlined.

Overtraining is the number-one mistake among bodybuilders who are trying to put on size, but who are failing to reach their potential. You have to be honest with yourself to recognize the fine line between pushing yourself maximally to complete each workout and pushing past that point into a catabolic state, excessively tearing down muscle.

For instance, especially during the "Three-Month Power Program" in Chapter 10, approach each set with focus and intensity. If you fail to reach your goal within that set, do not try to make up for that by adding more sets or exercises.

HAZARD #2: SACRIFICING FORM FOR REPS
DETOUR: USE PERFECT FORM

Bodybuilders often get so focused on completing their target reps that they begin to sacrifice form. If you're doing this, you're

CHAPTER ELEVEN

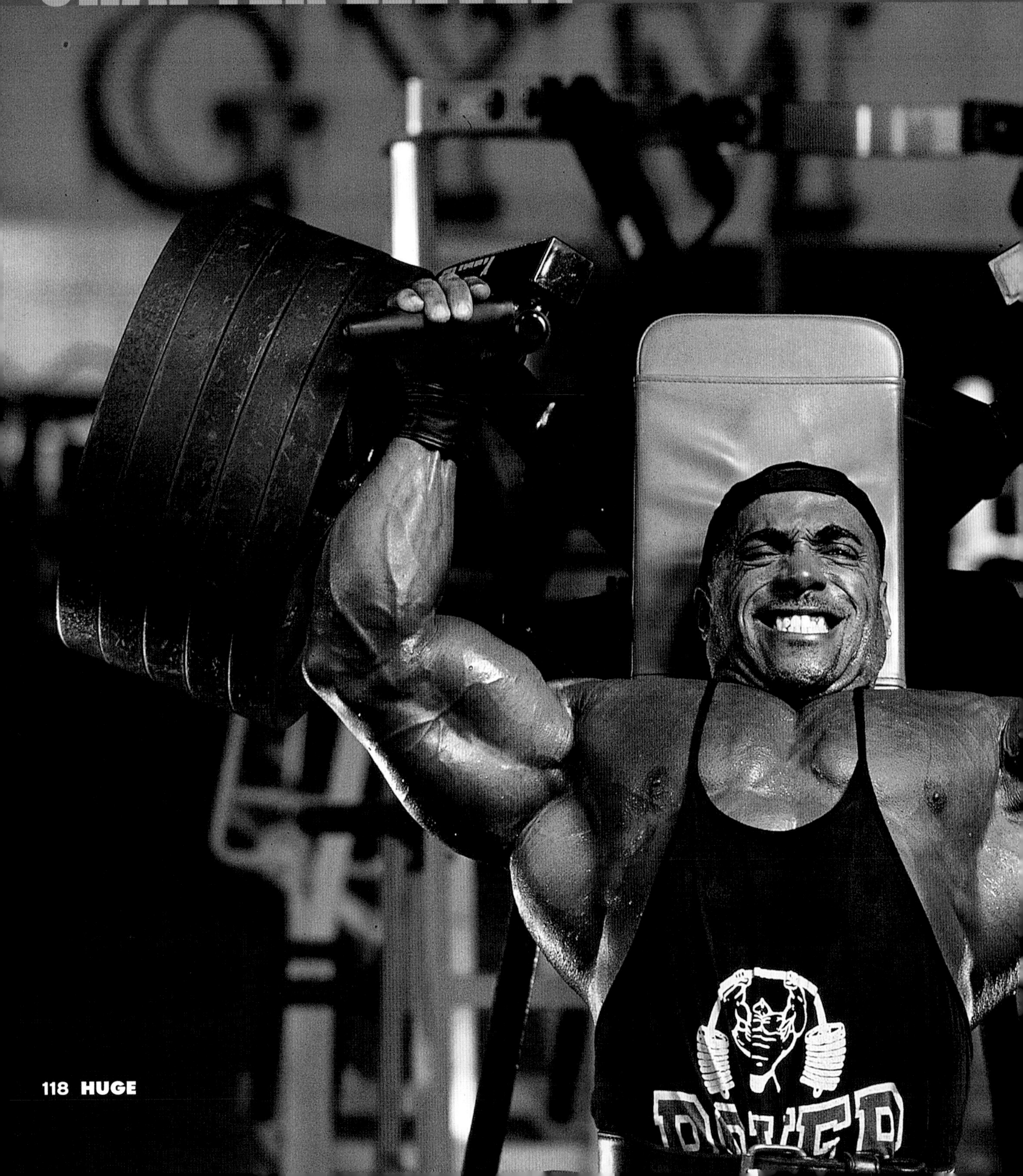

creating an environment for injury, and you're pushing past the bounds of ideal growth, potentially undermining your efforts.

Using perfect form achieves two goals: It helps you prevent injury and it provides a guideline for understanding when you have reached failure. If you cannot complete a rep with perfect form, then stop. You have already given your body the maximum load it can handle.

HAZARD #3: INATTENTION WHILE TRAINING
DETOUR: STAY FOCUSED AT THE GYM

Inattention can take many forms. Too many gym rats treat their workouts as the biggest social event of the day. Although it's obvious that you should try to avoid these folks, that's not always easy. It's up to you to set boundaries. Don't

During the three-month power phase, approach each set with focus and intensity.

feel inclined to indulge those who would sabotage your workout. Put on your game face and perform your next set, even if they're still yapping at you.

Of even more concern are the ways your own inattention can derail your workout. While performing a set, stay in the moment. You should never be thinking about your last rep, except when you're performing it. Keep your attention staunchly focused on the rep you're performing. Concentrate on contracting during the positive phase; feel your muscle stretching during the negative.

HAZARD #4: EGO TRAINING
DETOUR: TRAIN PROPERLY FOR YOUR GOALS

In Chapter 10, we carefully explained the difference between training for gaining muscle and for increasing strength. Of tantamount importance in this distinction is recognizing the role of the "pump." Bodybuilders often feel they can't grow if they don't get a pump. That's not true. Growth comes from stressing muscle fibers and encouraging them to repair themselves, not from engorging muscle tissues with blood. Bodybuilders confuse these principles because pumping your muscles makes you feel and look as though you're maximizing them.

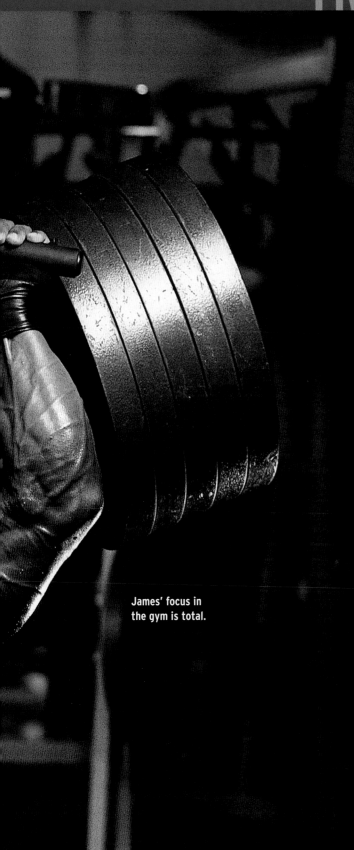
James' focus in the gym is total.

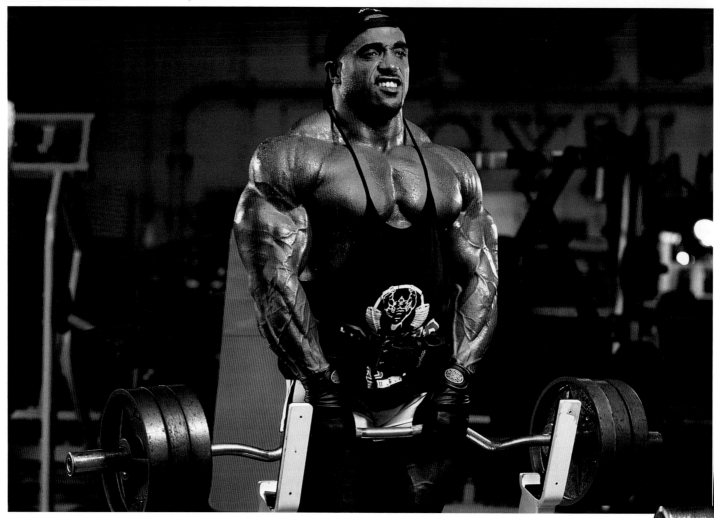

While doing a power program like that in Chapter 10, stay with your strength training on days designated for that. Accept that you are doing as much as you can for muscle growth by following the *FLEX* power protocol and that working to pump up your muscles at the end of a power session will only undercut your goals.

HAZARD #5: LAX NUTRITION HABITS
DETOUR: BE RIGOROUS WITH YOUR NUTRITION
As a bodybuilder, you have to devote only an hour or so a day to your training. The remainder of the day, you should focus on nutrition.

Many bodybuilders get sloppy with their nutrition, skipping a meal here or there, sometimes missing out on as many as 10 meals a week. If you want to make size gains, schedule meals and eat whether you're hungry or not. Waiting until you're hungry means you aren't providing your body with a steady stream of nutrients; your body won't have a continual supply of building blocks at its disposal for ultimate muscle growth. Work to adhere rigorously to a reasonable bodybuilding nutrition plan.

It is particularly important that you follow your post-workout nutrition protocol. Consume as many as 100 grams of simple carbs, with up to 50 grams of protein, a few minutes after your workout. Then, within the next hour or so, take in a full meal of protein, complex carbs and healthy fats.

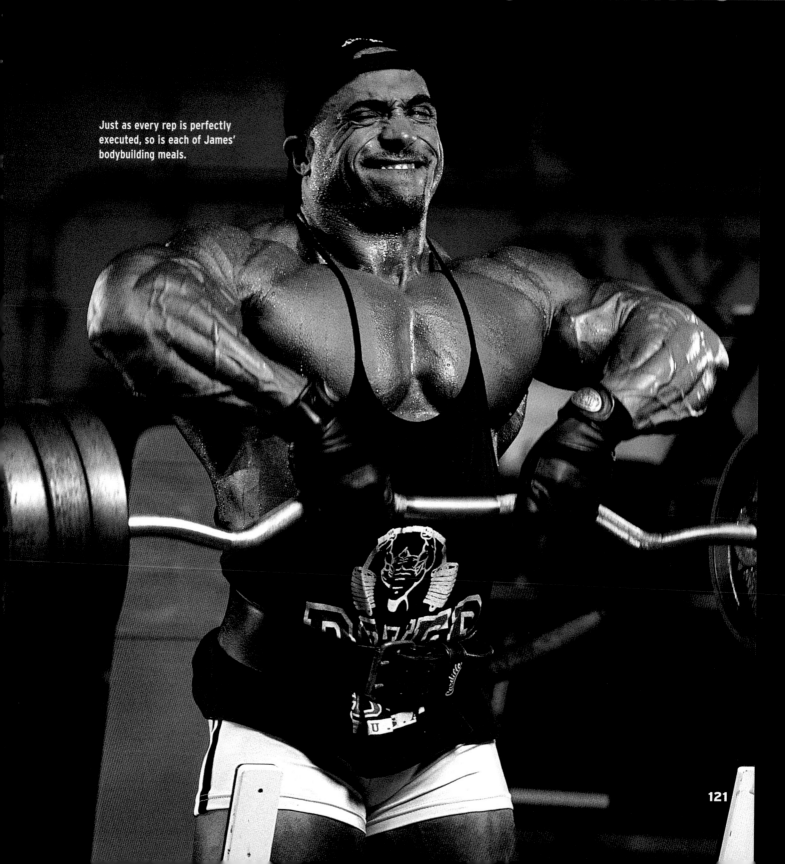

Just as every rep is perfectly executed, so is each of James' bodybuilding meals.

CHAPTER ELEVEN

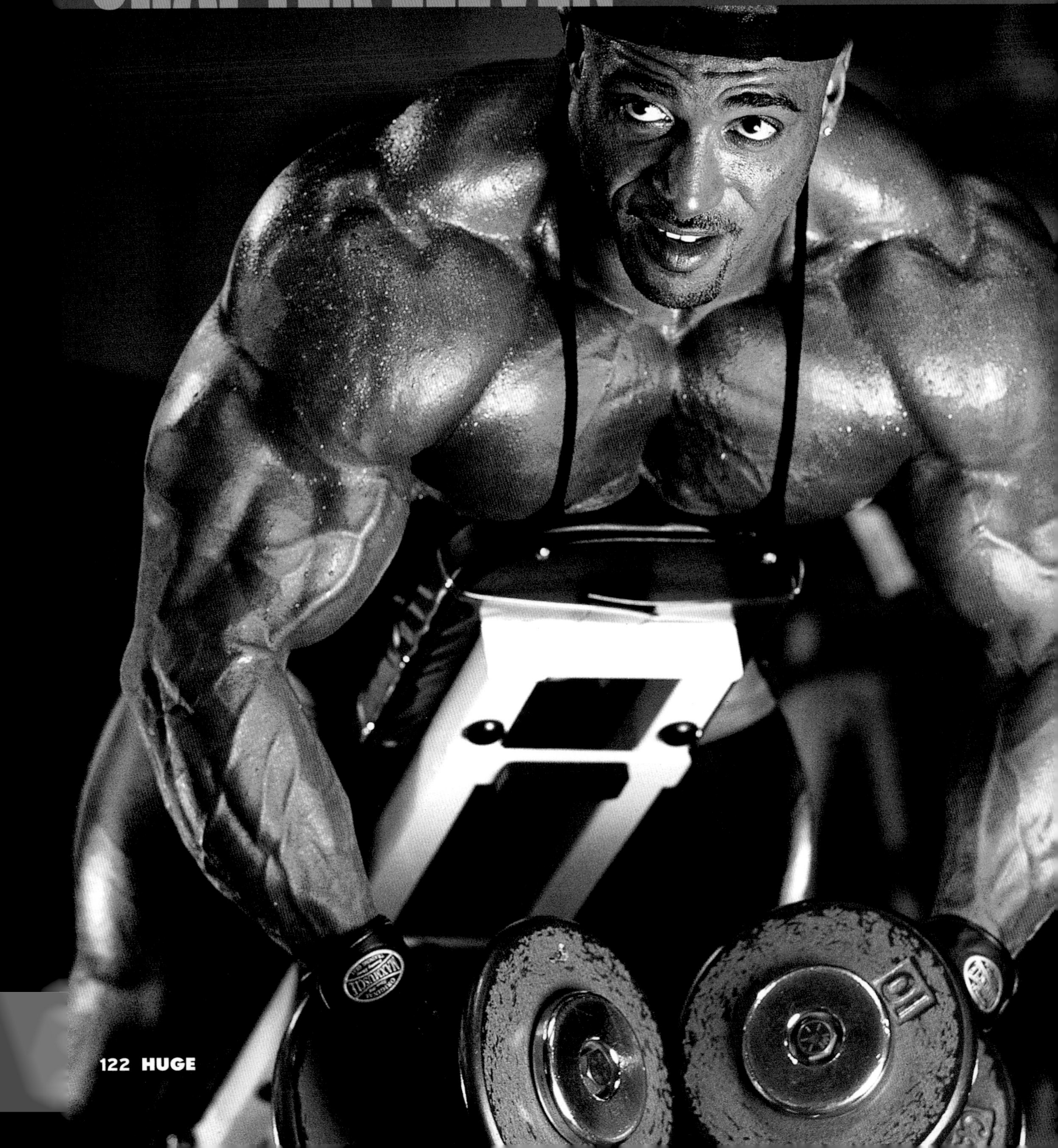

HAZARD #6: INATTENTION TO RECOVERY
DETOUR: BE MINDFUL OF RECOVERY

Nothing is more relaxing after a hard day of working and training than to hang out with friends and have a few beers, right? Who cares that you have to get up early and do it all again the next day? Well, your body does. Even if you don't feel it the way others seem to, ravaging yourself with late-night partying or simply not getting proper rest eventually takes its toll on your physique.

The average person needs eight hours of sleep a night, and bodybuilders are more than average. You may need nine or more hours of sleep a night for maximal growth. You may be functional or feel good on less, but take a few weeks to get a little more sleep and see if you don't notice physique gains coming more easily. Add an hour or so to the time you spend in bed each night or, even better, add an afternoon nap, if possible.

Also, be mindful that recovery goes beyond sleep. Relaxation activities and supplementation can have a major impact on your ability to recover. Relaxation can be focused (massage, acupuncture, yoga or meditation) or indirect (watching TV or simply spending a relaxing evening at home).

HAZARD #7: INCONSISTENCY
DETOUR: STICK TO YOUR PLAN

Consistency is at the core of sports performance, and nowhere is that more true than in bodybuilding. In the iron sport, consistency encompasses all aspects — training, nutrition, supplementation and recovery. To get the most from your bodybuilding regimen, chart out all the details of your day, then stick to the plan. Train on your training days, rest on your rest days. Eat your meals when you're supposed to. Above all, make certain that your expectations of yourself are reasonable so that you will adhere to them.

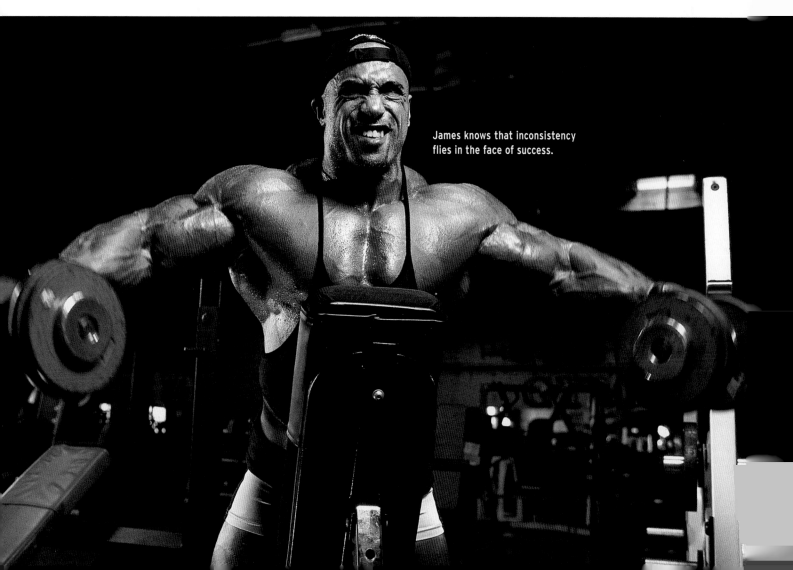

James knows that inconsistency flies in the face of success.

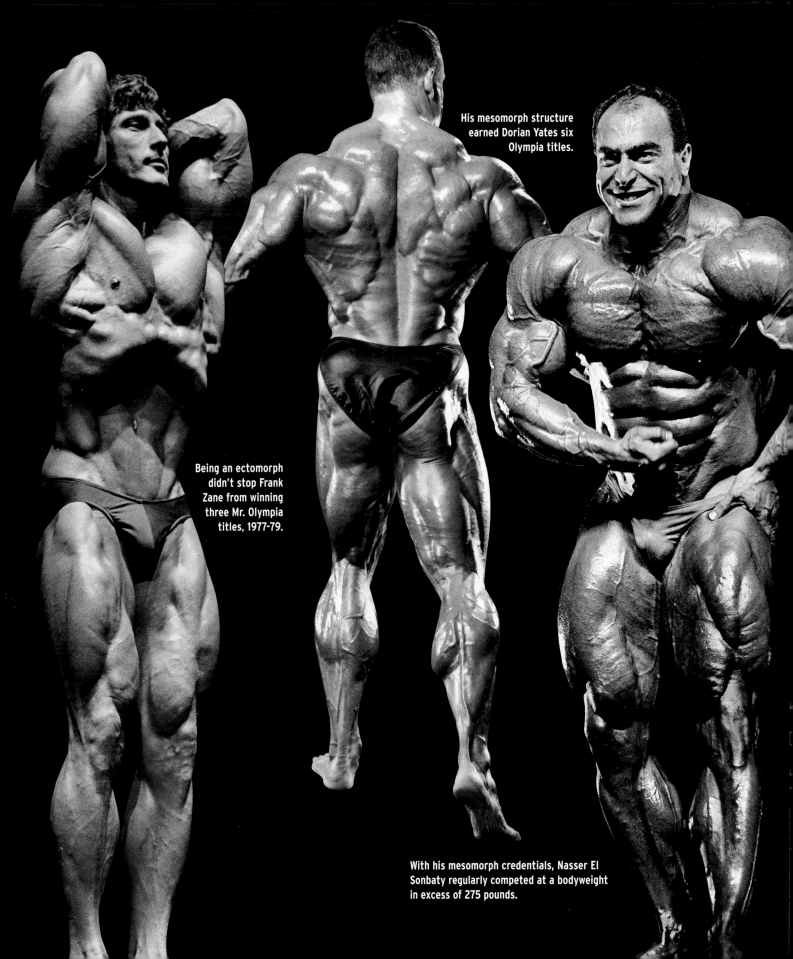

Being an ectomorph didn't stop Frank Zane from winning three Mr. Olympia titles, 1977-79.

His mesomorph structure earned Dorian Yates six Olympia titles.

With his mesomorph credentials, Nasser El Sonbaty regularly competed at a bodyweight in excess of 275 pounds.

Know Your BODYTYPE

Whatever your genetic disposition, you can still maximize your muscular potential

Secret revealed: Spend years doing what Dorian Yates does and with the same intensity, but the odds are still greater than a million to one against looking like the six-time Mr. Olympia. The reason for this is represented by three letters: DNA. DNA is your genetic blueprint, and it predetermines such factors as your skeletal structure, the shape of your muscles and your propensity for gaining lean mass. The bad news is you can't alter your DNA any more than you can choose your biological parents.

The good news is virtually everyone, regardless of genetics, can make dramatic physical changes by following bodybuilding practices. Furthermore, if you understand which factors you can't change, you can then work to maximize those you can.

GOOD GENES

What exactly are the ideal bodybuilding genetic characteristics? Obviously, first and foremost is the hormonal and physiological ability to gain muscle mass easily. If you pack on lean pounds quicker than others of similar size and experience do, odds are you have better-than-average genetics. At the same time, you may be the type who doesn't gain fat easily. If you've always been quite lean, regardless of your diet plan, it's a fair bet you have at least an average metabolism.

It's not enough to be capable of easily adding muscle and deflecting fat. Proper structure counts, too. The prototypical ideal bodybuilding anatomy includes wide clavicles and a narrow pelvis (narrow hipbones tend to also mean a narrow waist when fat-free), as well as long full muscles with short tendon attachments.

SOMATOTYPING

There are three widely accepted physique categories called somatotypes: endomorph, ectomorph and mesomorph. Endomorphs have large bones, wide hips (and waists), short muscles, and they gain fat easily. Ectomorphs are small boned but have long limbs, narrow shoulders and hips (and waists) and are naturally thin. Mesomorphs are naturally muscular with larger-than-average bones and rib cages.

If you're a male with wrists smaller than seven inches, your bones are slight, which means you're probably an ectomorph.

What follows are broad training guidelines for the three different somatotypes.

ENDOMORPH TRAINING Those who have a naturally slow metabolism need to emphasize restricting and burning calories. Cardio should be a regular part of your program. Weight training is not the time to lose fat. High reps do not burn appreciatively more calories than low reps, so stick to moderate reps and focus on gaining muscle mass. The added muscle itself utilizes more calories than fat does. Because endomorphs often have less energy than others do, don't severely restrict carbohydrates.

ECTOMORPH TRAINING In contrast to endomorphs, most ectomorphs have more than enough energy. Many of them are like walking and talking power plants. If you're an ectomorph, your key to gaining weight is to both consume more calories (especially protein) and use less energy. Extreme ectomorphs should avoid all cardio work. Keep your work-

The good news is virtually everyone, regardless of genetics, can make dramatic physical changes by following bodybuilding practices.

If your wrists are larger than seven and a half inches, you're big boned and likely an endomorph or mesomorph. However, if you're a mesomorph with relatively small bones you're in the best of all worlds, as full muscles swelling from small joints look most impressive. On the other hand, having large bones is somewhat of a tradeoff, as you probably gain mass more easily than others do but tend to have wider hips and less of a swell to your muscles.

By the time you reach your 20s, your natural shape may be obscured by years of activity or inactivity and a good or bad diet. To determine your somatotype, think back to your childhood and teenage years. Were you naturally chubby (endomorph), thin (ectomorph) or muscular (mesomorph)? Few people fit entirely into any category. Unless you were the "fat kid," "skinny kid" or "buff kid" growing up, odds are you possess qualities from two somatotypes. What's important is realizing what tendencies you have. Knowing which somatotype(s) you are most associated with will help you better formulate a training program and diet to maximize your strengths and minimize your weaknesses.

outs short, heavy and intense.

Focus on low reps for the basic compound lifts (e.g., squats, deadlifts and incline presses). Don't train any bodypart other than calves or abdominals more than once every four days (once every five days may be ideal). Try to get at least eight hours of sleep per night, and consume an easily digestible protein meal (such as a protein shake) two hours before bedtime.

MESOMORPH TRAINING Finally, we come to the lucky minority who grow easily. You chosen ones seem to accumulate muscle cells by merely looking at barbells. However, contrary to appearances, you haven't transcended the same rules of diet and training that govern all mortals. The natural inclination of mesomorphs (and, indeed, any trainers who start to make good gains) is to do more of the same. You think that if 12 sets for biceps are working, 20 sets must be better. Wrong! Overtraining (and overdoing anything) is the bane of the mesomorph. Note that many pro bodybuilders (often extreme mesomorphs) work each bodypart only once per

Zane's career was a study in perseverance.

In the gym and in his diet, Zane
became an expert on Zane.

week. Mesomorphs should combine high intensity with moderate volume.

STRUCTURAL IMPROVEMENTS

Mesomorphs have it made, and ectomorphs come in a close second. It's much easier for a naturally skinny individual to pack on 50 pounds of muscle than it is for an easy gainer to achieve a dramatic hip-to-shoulder differential. Consider the plight of the endomorph, cursed with wide hips and narrow shoulders. Almost anyone can add mass with enough effort and time, but that boxy endomorph can never stretch his clavicles or shrink his pelvic girdle.

Although bones cannot be altered, your V taper can be dramatically improved by accentuating side delts and upper-lat development and de-emphasizing hip and oblique muscles. Intermediate and advanced trainers with narrow shoulders should place special focus on side delts by performing two exercises for this area: side laterals and upright rows with a shoulder-width grip. Do three or four sets of each movement. You may want to perform at least one of these lifts first in your shoulder routine, when your energy and focus are greatest.

You probably don't need any encouragement to train your upper lats, as this is not a commonly neglected area. However, be aware that pullups or pulldowns to the front place particular emphasis on the high lat area around your underarms, thus accentuating your width when viewed from the front. Again, consider doing pullups or front pulldowns first in your back routine.

Thankfully, you can't expand your pelvis through exercise. However, you can grow the muscles on the outside of your hips. For this reason, if you have wide hips and sufficiently large thighs, you may want to avoid heavy squats and medium or low reps for any hip abduction exercises. Likewise, if you have a wide waist, you should do only high reps (20 or more) for oblique exercises like side bends and twists, or avoid training the "sidelines" entirely. Instead, shift the focus to maximizing your shoulders and upper lats.

MUSCLE LENGTHENING

Another crucial genetic factor for your bodybuilding success is the shape and length of your muscles. This is true not only because bodyparts that fill out your limbs and torso appear most impressive, but also because longer muscles with shorter tendons have greater leverage, making them stronger and generally larger. Understand that muscle length is relative.

THE LOWER ROAD

The accompanying chart lists the best exercises for hitting your "lowers." (Bodyparts like chest and shoulders are left off the list because there's little advantage to targeting the low insertions.) Give the prescribed exercises greater focus in your program. For example, if your gastrocnemius muscles are bunched high up on your lower legs, do more seated calf raises, which target your soleus, a muscle that travels the length of your calves. Instead of performing three or four sets of seated calf raises, try six sets and place them first in your routine. Likewise, if you have high lats, do cable rows and one-arm dumbbell rows in each back routine, because these lifts stretch your lower lats. You cannot turn especially high calves into bulging diamonds or latissimus dorsi with high attachments into low sweeping wings, but with concentrated effort, you can make noticeable improvements to your muscle shape.

In the case of thighs and calves, the lifts focus on specific muscles within a group: the vastus medialis and soleus, respectively. The other exercises target the bottom insertion of a muscle. You can't truly isolate areas within an individual muscle. For example, you cannot make only your lower biceps grow. However, you can focus slightly more stress on a muscle's lowest area with either a strong stretch (as in preacher curls) or strong contraction (as in triceps kickbacks).

LOWER-MUSCLE EXERCISES

BODYPART	EXERCISE
Lower biceps	Preacher curls
Lower triceps	Kickbacks
Lower lats	Cable rows
	One-arm dumbbell rows
Lower thighs	Hack squats
	Leg extensions
Lower calves	Seated calf raises

Although bones cannot be altered, your V taper can be dramatically improved by accentuating side delts and upper-lat development.

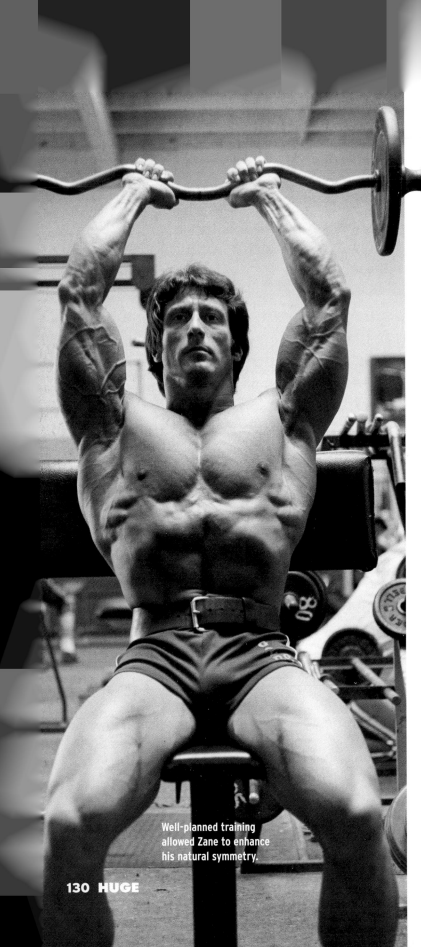

Well-planned training allowed Zane to enhance his natural symmetry.

Bodybuilder A has long arm bones, but a wide gap between his flexed biceps and his arm joints, and bodybuilder B has short arm bones that overflow with flexed sinew. A's biceps are considered short, even though they may be longer than B's. Shorter individuals tend to have fuller muscles in relation to their smaller frames, whereas many tall trainers have difficulty filling out their limbs.

You cannot appreciably alter the length of your muscles, but you can focus on the lower area of a muscle group or a

Unless you're battling for a pro card or a pro win, it's unlikely you'll be held back by your skeletal or muscular structure.

muscle. One way to do this is by fully stretching each body-part before and after training it. Among other benefits, stretching will help your muscles achieve their maximum length. You should also choose those exercises that place special emphasis on the lower area of a muscle or the lowest muscle of a bodypart (see "The Lower Road").

GENES AND YOU

Many experts say genetics are the most important factor in bodybuilding. This may be true when it comes to describing the differences between you and Mr. Olympia or even why one man finishes first and another last in the Mr. O. However, the simple truth is unless you're battling for a pro card or a pro win, it's unlikely you'll be held back by your skeletal or muscular structure or the rate at which you gain mass or lose fat. With the proper training and nutrition and enough rest and patience, almost anyone can transform his physique dramatically. Sure, the overwhelming odds are you'll never be Mr. Olympia, but then only one person on the planet ever is at one time. What's important is understanding your genetic strengths and weaknesses, and using this knowledge to achieve the muscular proportionate body you desire.

It took hard training and great genetics for Ronnie Coleman to craft one of the best backs in the history of the sport.

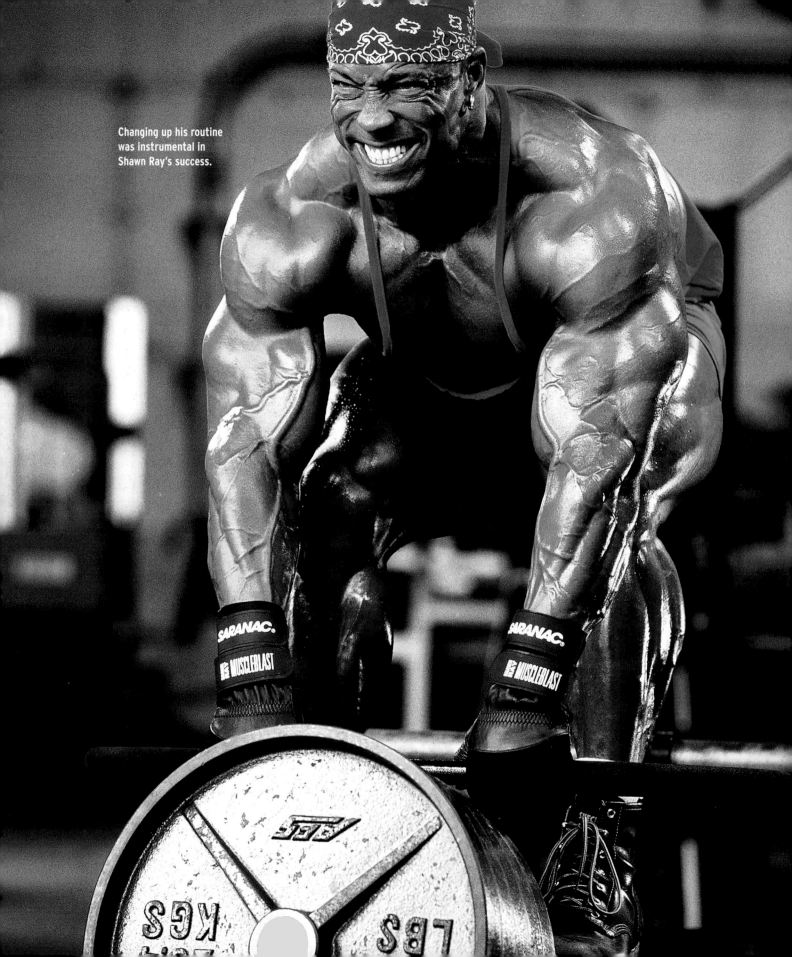

Changing up his routine
was instrumental in
Shawn Ray's success.

The NEXT STEP

This mix-it-up training program will lead to crazy gains in 13 weeks

You must be tired by now. And stronger. You've experienced the size gains of "Mass Attack" (see Chapter 3), and for the last three months, you have been lugging through an ambitious 13-week power routine (see Chapter 10). That Power Surge phase was designed to rewire your central nervous system to master your body's response to intensely heavy loads. You also learned how to mentally overcome the pain threshold and take your physical capabilities further than you ever have before.

The power phase made you mightier. Now it's time to get meatier.

That moaning you hear is your muscles, fatigued but hungry — hungry to grow. They're begging for the exact stimulus in the precise sequence required to begin their journey to big town. The following 13-week segment is exactly the kick start your muscles need. Your body is primed to add mass. It's grow time!

ROUTINES THAT AREN'T ROUTINE

As we've lectured endlessly, the premise of the program outlined in this book is that you cannot increase muscle mass effectively if you only try to build muscle mass. You must also increase strength. To do that, you must train differently than you did to increase muscle mass.

Your inclination at this point may be to jump back into a bodybuilding-style pump routine, where you grind out eight to 12 reps for every set. Trust us — that's not the best approach. Instead, this 13-week program gives you elements lacking in most workout plans. The 13 weeks are split into five different segments and are explained in detail as you work your way through this chapter.

To start, we're asking you to take a week off, far away from the weights. "Huh?" you may be asking. "FLEX wants me to stay out of the gym?"

Yeah, dude. And not because you wear those too-tight purple Lycra shorts and leave pools of sweat on the flat bench (if you do, stop it). It's because your entire body needs to settle down after all that volume from the power surge phase. We're calling it "active rest," so don't lounge on the couch and stare at Jennifer Love Hewitt movies all day. Don't lift, but don't stay sedentary either. Play softball, throw a Frisbee, get lucky. Active rest, get it?

Then, after a week away from the gym, we're asking you to do something that may seem kind of pencilnecky at first: circuit training. But bear with us, the rationale is explained later on. After two weeks of circuitry, you'll get into what we call a "back to bodybuilding" segment. These are more traditional three-sets-of-10-reps types of workouts. You'll do this during weeks four through seven. And you'll enjoy it — a lot. Your body will never be more ready for this type of lifting than after its circuit reconditioning.

Then, it's back to power surging, but only for another two weeks. These challenging workouts will toss in high- and low-rep work. There's plenty of volume and variation to really fool your muscles — and Mother Nature — into making you a better monster.

After two weeks in power mode, you'll return to the bodybuilding fundamentals and have a pumpin' good time in weeks 10 to 13. That's four weeks of good old bodybuilding in its more conventional form: three sets, eight to 15 reps, a hearty pump and long looks in a mirror. By that time, you should be impressing more than yourself.

Let's review the entire phase three.

Week 1: Active Rest
Weeks 2-3: Circuit Training
Weeks 4-7: Back to Bodybuilding
Weeks 8-9: Power to the People
Weeks 10-13: Fun with Fundamentals

On paper, it looks insane. But give this 13-week Crazy Gains program the attention and respect it deserves. You'd be nuts not to. Now, let's look at this phase segment by segment.

Week 1: Active Rest

In some ways, this is the hardest part of the entire program, as we ask bodybuilders to do the one thing they hate: Stay out of the gym for an entire week. Don't even pick up a weight.

After the 13-week power phase, you need to give your body a rest — your joints, tendons, ligaments and mind, as well as your muscles. Don't worry, you won't lose a whit of your newly acquired poundages. In fact, it's been well documented by sports scientists, successful strength coaches and bodybuilders themselves that these gains are maintained better by resting.

Now, what precisely does "active rest" mean? Basically, it means to be physical, but in ways that promote recovery rather than further muscle breakdown; it means to exercise, but lightly, and to keep away from the weights.

Play basketball or participate in another favorite sport. Include a few moderate cardio sessions — no more than three or four easy sessions of 20 to 30 minutes.

The goal is not to burn bodyfat (that will come in the final workout phase of the program), but to get your blood pumping and give your body both a different and a gentler form of physical stimulation. This is also a good time to experiment with other more exotic types of "rest" activities, such as stretching, yoga or massage.

Weeks 2-3: Circuit Training

You may have done circuit training in the past. It means moving quickly from one exercise to the next; doing a set of one exercise, then moving to an entirely different exercise, without resting in between. It's high volume, low intensity (see "Circuit Training" charts for details).

Do circuit training four days per week for two weeks. Think of it as retraining your circuitry to prepare your muscles for pure bodybuilding workouts.

Believe it or not, nothing primes your body for a shift — whether from a strength-power phase or from scratch or a layoff — to serious muscle-building workouts like circuit training. Yes, these workouts are different. Not what you'd expect to see in FLEX. And not the most exciting or challenging workouts. But, take it from us, this approach works.

The purpose of these two weeks is to provide another step

up in exercise volume. Each training day, do four different circuits, twice in the prescribed order. Each circuit comprises five exercises, for 40 sets per workout four times a week. That's a lot of sets. However, although the volume is high, the intensity is low, just perfect for preparing you for weeks four to seven.

CIRCUIT TRAINING
MONDAY AND THURSDAY:
LOWER-BODY EMPHASIS

CIRCUIT ONE
Leg presses
Toe presses on a leg-press machine
V-grip pulldowns
Upright rows
Hyperextensions

CIRCUIT TWO
Leg curls
Machine or freestanding front squats
Leg extensions
Seated calf raises
Reverse crunches

CIRCUIT THREE
Hack squats
Dumbbell side laterals
Stiff-leg deadlifts
Standing heel raises
Forward crunches

CIRCUIT FOUR
Barbell or dumbbell lunges
Triceps pressdowns
Dumbbell shrugs
Barbell curls
Rope crunches

CIRCUIT TRAINING
TUESDAY AND FRIDAY:
UPPER-BODY EMPHASIS

CIRCUIT ONE
Overhead presses
Close-grip pulldowns
Seated dumbbell curls
Dips
Hyperextensions

CIRCUIT TWO
Bench presses
Chest-supported rows
Calf raises
Cross-bench dumbbell pullovers
Twisting crunches

CIRCUIT THREE
V-grip low-pulley rows
Overhead triceps extensions
Seated calf raises
Leg curls
Barbell shrugs

CIRCUIT FOUR
Close-grip cambered-bar bench presses
Cable rows
Pec-deck flyes
Deep squats with one-half bodyweight
Incline dumbbell curls

You will definitely not be getting a serious pump (if you are, you're missing the point). Use roughly 40-50% of your one-rep max (1RM) weight for these exercises and do 15 reps per set over the course of about 30 seconds in a rhythmic controlled fashion. Rest only 30 seconds, then hit the next exercise in the circuit. Try to focus on the clock instead of on how many reps you're performing. Each successive set targets a different bodypart, allowing the just-trained bodypart to rest, while you continue to keep the blood pumping, the heart working and the calories burning.

We've listed several examples of circuits, but we realize that you may not be able to use this specific equipment in a regular gym environment. Feel free to substitute or change the order of exercises. The key elements of the program are high volume, low intensity and a large variety of exercises.

Don't try to see how many reps you can do each set; the goal is to keep moving and to focus on perfect form and on feeling the pump in the appropriate muscle group. This period is about progressive reconditioning that helps rejuvenate your nervous system, your joints and connective tissue, your muscles and your mind.

It also enhances your anaerobic and aerobic fitness base, ultimately and optimally preparing your body for its continuing foray into the realm of ever-increasing levels of overload and muscle growth.

NOTES

■ *Prior to each workout, warm up for five or six minutes on a bike or treadmill.*

■ *Perform three sets of 15 reps (at 40-50% of your one-rep max) for each exercise.*

■ *When you've completed one set of each of the five exercises in a circuit, rest two minutes.*

■ *Run through each circuit twice total.*

■ *For ab work and hyperextensions (where no weight resistance is involved), simply complete the appropriate reps.*

■ *Based on preference or practicality, substitute exercises, as long as you are hitting the same muscle groups.*

Weeks 4-7: Back to Bodybuilding

At last! Back to conventional bodybuilding workouts and mind-blowing pumps. In this segment, work out four times a week, training each bodypart once. Cut back on the number of exercises, sets and reps, but increase the poundages and the intensity to stimulate maximum muscle growth.

For each exercise, determine a weight with which you can perform one more rep than called for, using absolutely perfect form. After the appropriate warm-up, perform all your sets with that weight. For the first set, stop at the specified number of reps, even if you feel you can complete another rep or two with perfect form. After resting two minutes (three minutes between squats, leg presses, deadlifts and other heavy compound exercises),

Increase poundages and intensity to stimulate maximum muscle growth.

perform your second set, again stopping at the specified number of reps. For your third set, complete as many reps as you can with stellar form. Once there is a break of any kind in exercise form, that set is over. If you complete the specified number of reps for all the required sets, increase the

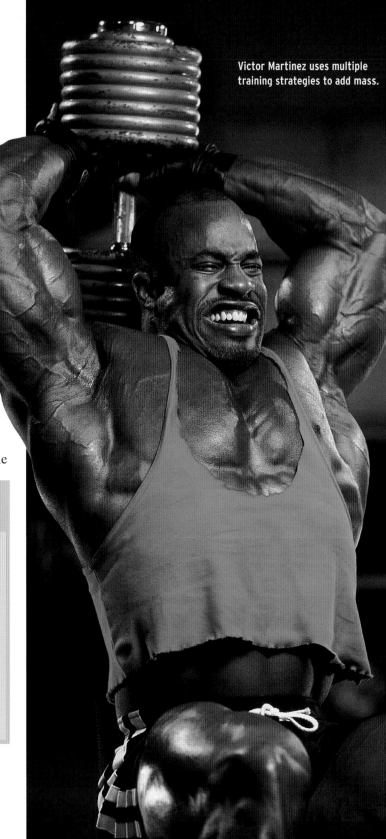

Victor Martinez uses multiple training strategies to add mass.

MONDAY: QUADS AND CALVES

EXERCISE	SETS	REPS
QUADS		
Hyperextensions	2*	15
Knee extensions	3†	10
Hack squats	3†	10
Smith machine or barbell lunges	3	10
Leg presses	3	10
CALVES		
Donkey heel raises	3	15
Seated heel raises	3	20

*Hyperextensions are performed as a safety factor to warm up the lower back prior to heavy leg work.
† Warm up with two light sets of 20 reps.

TUESDAY: CHEST AND BICEPS

EXERCISE	SETS	REPS
CHEST		
Low-incline (10-degree) dumbbell presses	3*	10
45-degree incline dumbbell presses	3	10
Parallel-bar dips	3	8
Cable crossovers	3	10
BICEPS		
90-degree preacher curls	3*	8
Standing alternate dumbbell curls	3	8
Barbell reverse curls	3	12

Warm up with two light sets of 20 reps.

THURSDAY: BACK, HAMSTRINGS AND ABS

EXERCISE	SETS	REPS
BACK		
Hyperextensions	2	15
Deadlifts	3*	6
Dumbbell rows	2	6
Bent barbell rows (overhand grip)	3*	10
Close-grip pulldowns	3	10
HAMSTRINGS		
Leg curls	3*	8
Stiff-leg deadlifts	3	12
ABS		
Forward crunches superset with	3	20
Reverse crunches	3	20

Warm up with two light sets of 20 reps.

You should adopt perfect form for all reps to achieve maximum muscular response.

weight by 5% or so for your next workout. Prior to all workouts, warm up for five or six minutes on a bike or treadmill.

Weeks 8-9: Power to the People

After four weeks of pump-style bodybuilding work and the diet to support it (see "A Sane Diet Leads to Crazy Gains" at the end of this chapter), you'll be sporting a fuller look. Let's not forget how you got to this point — power, baby. For two weeks, take a break from your bodybuilding-style workouts and return to heavier weights for fewer reps.

Going back to the strength-power approach should be a productive mental and physiological change; it should also generate more enthusiasm as well as increased strength when this two-week period is over. The key is low-rep sets of five reps — which would equate to 85% of your 1RM. Understand that when you work a muscle at the intensity of 85% of its 1RM, you generate the optimum strength and muscle gains. But you can only work at that level for short periods, hence the two-week regimen. In order to maintain this intensity of effort, train only three times a week, hitting each bodypart once a week (turn the page for your prescribed workouts).

Even though you are working with heavy poundages, you should adopt perfect form for all reps to achieve maximum muscular response. Rest at least three minutes and up to five between five-rep sets. Prior to all workouts, warm up for five or six minutes on a bike or treadmill.

FRIDAY: SHOULDERS AND TRICEPS

EXERCISE	SETS	REPS
SHOULDERS		
Seated dumbbell presses	3*	10*
Seated Smith machine presses	2	10
Bent dumbbell laterals	3	12
Standing side laterals	3	12
TRICEPS		
Close-grip bench presses	3†	10
Rope pressdowns	3	10
Seated dumbbell overhead extensions	3	10

Warm up with two light sets of 20 reps, plus two light sets of 20 reps of dumbbell side laterals.
† *Warm up with two light sets of 20 reps.*

MONDAY:
QUADS, CALVES AND ABS

EXERCISE	SETS	REPS
QUADS		
Hyperextensions	2*	15
Barbell squats	5†	10, 5, 5, 5, 10
Leg presses	3	10, 5, 5
CALVES		
Standing calf raises	4	10, 5, 5, 5
ABS		
Forward crunches	3	15
superset with		
Reverse crunches	3	15

*Hyperextensions are performed as a safety factor to warm up the lower back prior to heavy leg work.
† Warm up with two light sets of 20 reps.

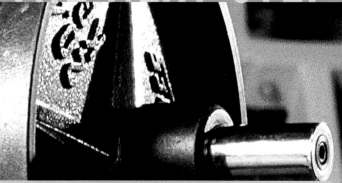

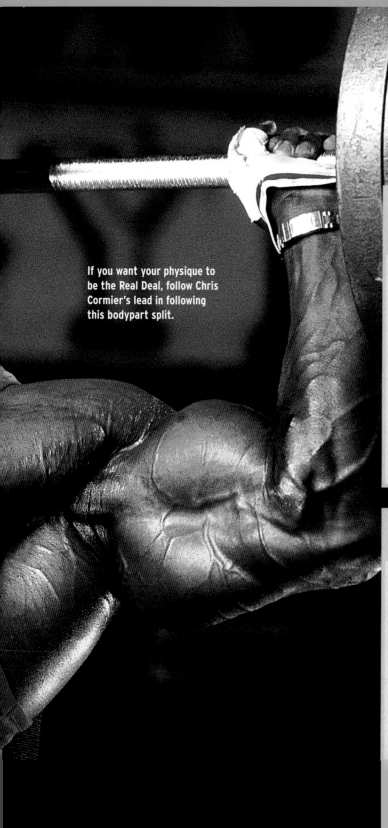

If you want your physique to be the Real Deal, follow Chris Cormier's lead in following this bodypart split.

WEDNESDAY:
CHEST, SHOULDERS AND TRICEPS

EXERCISE	SETS	REPS
CHEST		
Incline (30-degree) bench presses	3*	5
Flat-bench dumbbell presses	3	5
Incline (45-degree) dumbbell flyes	3	10
SHOULDERS		
Seated barbell presses	3†	5
One-arm cable lateral raises	3	15
TRICEPS		
Lying triceps extensions	3*	6
Triceps pushdowns	2	8

*Warm up with two light sets of 20 reps.
† Warm up with two light sets of 20 reps, plus two light sets of 20 reps of dumbbell side laterals.

FRIDAY:
BACK AND BICEPS

EXERCISE	SETS	REPS
BACK		
Hyperextensions	2*	15
Deadlifts	5†	10, 5, 5, 5, 10
Barbell rows	3	10, 5, 5
Close-grip pulldowns	3	8
BICEPS		
Barbell curls	3†	6
Preacher curls	2	8

*Hyperextensions are performed as a safety factor to warm up the lumbar region prior to back work.
† Warm up with two light sets of 20 reps.

Weeks 10-13: Fun with Fundamentals

To complete this training phase, we've scheduled four more weeks of higher volume work. This segment is designed to get the blood pumping and the muscle fibers expanding. You're back to training four times a week and, based on the previous nine weeks work, you should now be stronger and ready to apply even more stress to your greedy-for-growth muscle fibers.

As in weeks four through seven, for each exercise, determine a weight with which you can perform one more rep than called for, using absolutely perfect form. If you make the target reps, increase the weight by 5% for the next week. If you fail to make the target reps, stay with that poundage until you succeed. You will find that on some lifts and/or bodyparts, you will make faster progress than on others. The key is to stay with the 5% formula and don't cheat. In terms of rest between sets, take three minutes for larger bodyparts and two minutes for smaller bodyparts. Prior to all workouts, warm up for five or six minutes on a bike or treadmill.

MONDAY: LEGS

EXERCISE	SETS	REPS
QUADS		
Hyperextensions	2*	15
Barbell squats	4†	8
Leg presses	3	10
Front squats	3	10
HAMSTRINGS		
Leg curls	3†	10
Stiff-leg deadlifts	2	10
CALVES		
Standing calf raises	3	15
Toe presses on a leg-press machine	3	12

*Hyperextensions are performed as a safety factor to warm up the lower back prior to heavy leg work.
† Warm up with two light sets of 20 reps.

TUESDAY: ARMS

EXERCISE	SETS	REPS
TRICEPS		
Close-grip bench presses	4*	10
Overhead barbell extensions	3	10
Triceps pressdowns	2	12
Dips	2	10
BICEPS		
Barbell curls	3*	8
Incline dumbbell curls	3	8
90-degree preacher curls	2	10
Cambered-bar reverse curls	2	15

*Warm up with two light sets of 20 reps.

THURSDAY: CHEST AND SHOULDERS

EXERCISE	SETS	REPS
CHEST		
Decline bench presses	3*	10
Flat-bench flyes	3	8
Incline dumbbell presses	3	8
SHOULDERS		
Seated barbell presses	3*	8
Seated side laterals	3	8
Bent lateral raises	3	8
Shrugs	3	8

*Warm up with two light sets of 20 reps.

FRIDAY: BACK AND ABS

EXERCISE	SETS	REPS
BACK		
Hyperextensions	2*	15
Deadlifts	4†	8
Close-grip pulldowns	4	8
Barbell rows (overhand grip) or T-bar rows	4	8
ABS		
Forward crunches superset with	3	15
Reverse crunches	3	15

*Hyperextensions are performed as a safety factor to warm up the lumbar region prior to back work.
† Warm up with two light sets of 20 reps.

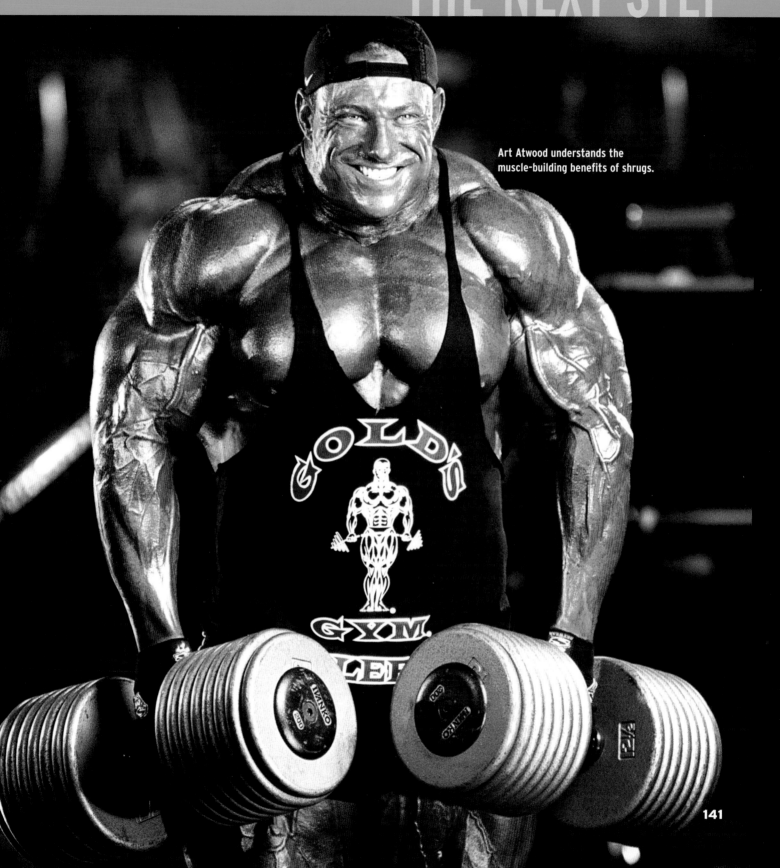

Art Atwood understands the muscle-building benefits of shrugs.

141

In addition to intense training, Tommi Thorvildsen focuses on intense eating.

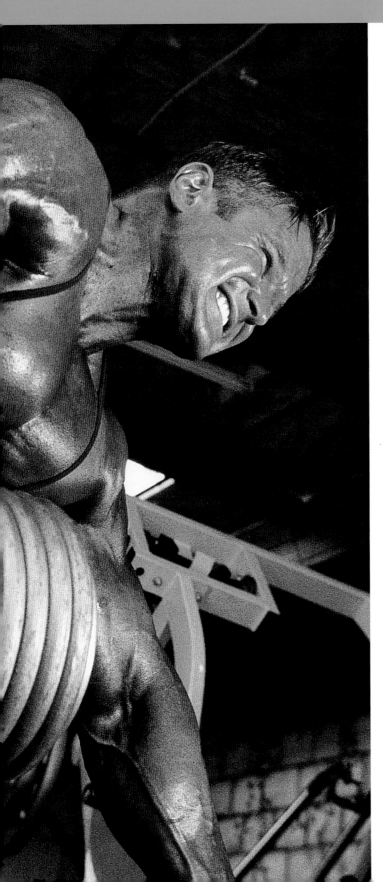

A SANE DIET LEADS TO CRAZY GAINS

To make crazy gains, you need proper nutritional support. Even during active-rest and circuit-training weeks, strive to continue to eat six meals a day. If you do not have a big appetite during those weeks, you might be unable to consume as many total calories as you otherwise could — that's OK. The emphasis should remain on how many meals you eat per day, rather than on how much you eat at each meal.

Focus on eating portions of rice, yams, potatoes and oatmeal at nearly every meal you eat.

As you get into this program, you may feel as though you're almost in a cutting phase because of the volume of training compared to the power phases. It's imperative that you always stay focused on the fact that this is still a gaining phase, and as such you need to concentrate on taking in the quality and quantity of nutrients you need for optimal muscle growth. Keep the following nutrition tips in mind.

■ Take in at least one gram of protein per pound of bodyweight per day. The protein should be fairly evenly distributed over your six meals.

■ Take in plenty of complex carbohydrates. Often, bodybuilders worry that too many carbs will make them fat. Don't. Complex carbs help you put on muscle mass. Focus on eating portions of rice, yams, potatoes and oatmeal at nearly every meal you eat. You might add a little bit of bodyfat (which you'll strip off in phase four), but this strategy will allow you to add more muscle mass than any diet that restricts carbohydrates.

■ Eat plenty of good fats. Use healthy oils, such as canola or olive, for cooking and seasoning. Include foods such as nuts, seeds, all-natural peanut butter and avocados to increase calories and healthy fats for recovery and well-being.

■ Drink plenty of water. Try to take in at least one gallon every day, in addition to other liquids.

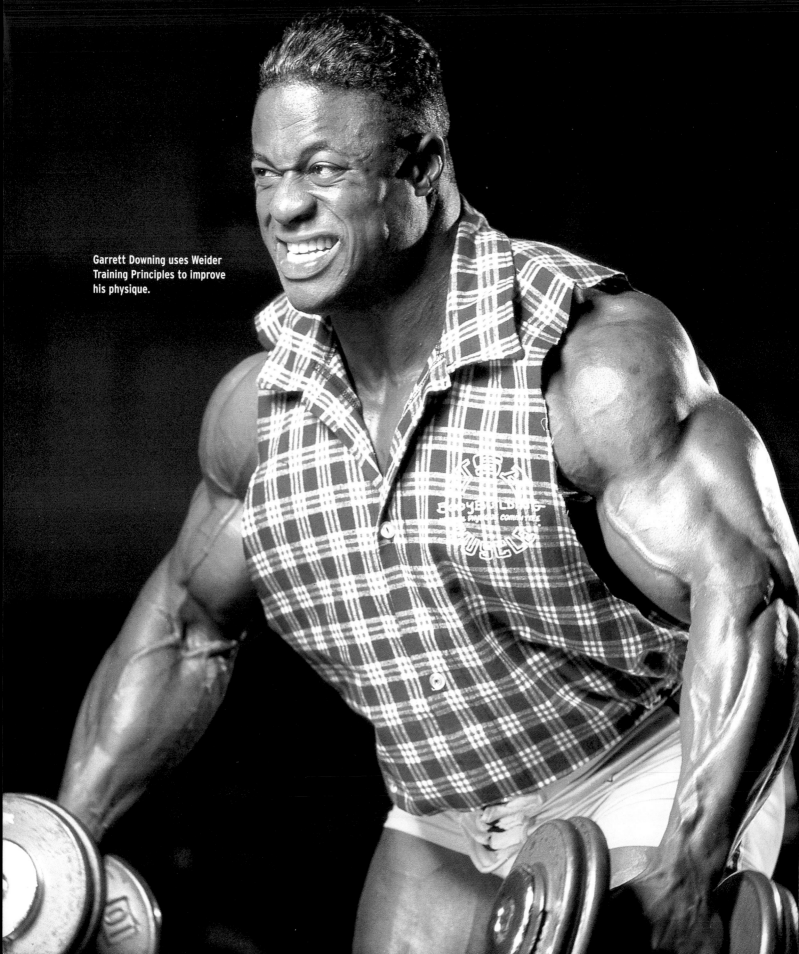

Rev Up
THE INTENSITY

Use the Weider Training Principles to accelerate your muscle gains

Based on the foundation you've laid down with the training programs in this book, you are primed to begin using certain Weider Training Principles in pursuit of increasing intensity and muscle mass.

Before getting to the guts of these techniques, a word of warning. These principles should be used sparingly. By increasing intensity, these principles take your body to the brink of overtraining. If you incorporate them too liberally, you will be stimulating more fatigue than is optimal for recovery and growth.

Limit the use of intensity techniques to the last set of a bodypart workout and apply them to only two bodyparts per workout. On the other hand, if your training is so intense and demanding that your body is already working at its upper limit, you might want to delay incorporating intensity techniques into your schedule. If that's the case, hold on to these training nuggets for later, and use them after you have had a chance to fully recover from the total body program. You can easily incorporate them into most routines.

The following are some of the most popular and effective intensity techniques, designed to help you add as much muscle mass as possible during this phase of your training.

WEIDER FORCED REPS TRAINING PRINCIPLE

Most bodybuilders already employ this intensity technique to

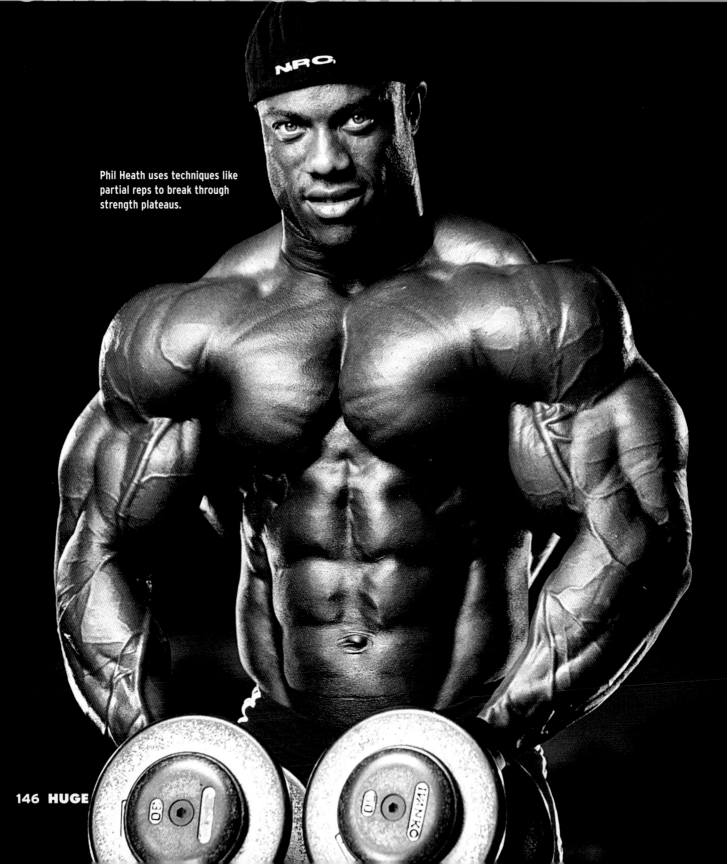

Phil Heath uses techniques like partial reps to break through strength plateaus.

a certain degree, but used more conscientiously, it can be even more effective. The forced reps principle requires a spotter to assist you when you can no longer perform another rep with perfect form. When this point is reached, the spotter gives just enough assistance to enable you to keep the weight moving yet maintain proper form. For instance, if you are performing 90-degree preacher bench curls with 70 pounds, you might be able to get only eight strict reps before failure kicks in. However, you probably still have enough strength left to perform two or three more reps with 40 or 50 pounds. By assisting you, the spotter "reduces" the amount of weight you must lift, so, in effect, you are reaching failure at 70 pounds, and then reaching it again with a "lower" weight. You are prolonging the set past the normal point of failure, increasing intensity on the muscle and therefore stimulating greater strength and growth.

To employ this technique, perform your regular set without assistance from your spotter. When you reach failure, go directly without resting into two or three forced reps. Maintain perfect form throughout your forced reps. Rather than cheating or breaking form, rely on your partner to absorb enough of the workload to enable you to maintain intensity and stay focused on your target muscle.

WEIDER REST-PAUSE TRAINING PRINCIPLE

The rest-pause principle, like the forced reps principle, allows you to prolong a set after the normal point of failure. Here's an example of how rest-pause works with Smith machine presses for shoulders. Say your target for this exercise is 10 reps. When you're unable to complete another rep with perfect form, rest the bar and, still seated in the machine, wait for 10 seconds. Then grip the bar and press out another rep with proper form.

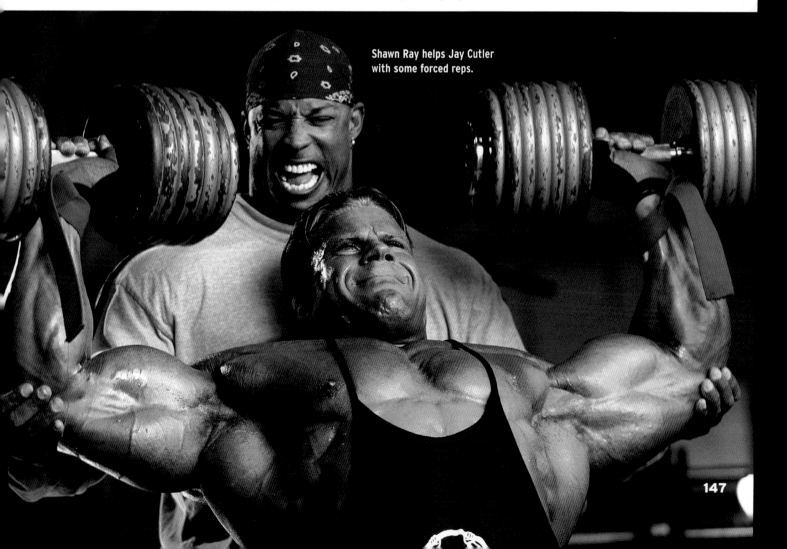

Shawn Ray helps Jay Cutler with some forced reps.

Take another 10-second rest, then do another full rep. You might be able to do a third rest-pause rep, but call it a day after that. This technique builds size and strength and is particularly useful for someone who does not have a training partner and therefore cannot attempt forced reps.

WEIDER NEGATIVE REPS TRAINING PRINCIPLE

The negative reps, or reverse-gravity, principle can be used for a variety of exercises, but its safest and most effective use occurs when you can maintain complete control of the negative portion of the movement, such as during machine and pulley exercises. As with forced reps, you must have a partner to assist you in using this technique.

Here's how to use this method when doing close-grip pulldowns. When you reach failure (the point at which you can no longer execute a rep with perfect form), you're ready to employ the negative reps principle. During the next rep,

The tendency with descending sets is to try to train with too much volume at the expense of fully taxing your target muscle. For this principle to be most effective, you must feel full fatigue from your working set, then transition quickly to your lower weight. You should reach fatigue with your lower weight by your second to fourth reps. If you are able to complete numerous reps at this lowered weight, the poundage is too light.

WEIDER PARTIAL REPS TRAINING PRINCIPLE

The strict interpretation of the partial reps principle involves doing half and three-quarter movements with poundages you cannot handle for full reps in order to break through sticking points. But here, we will focus on how to use partial reps at the end of a working set to prolong the set and the intensity of the exercise. After hitting failure, you will not have enough strength to complete a full rep, but you will have the strength

Limit intensity technique usage to the last set for a bodypart and apply them to only two bodyparts per workout.

have your training partner help you lift the weight stack so that the grip handle is against your chest. From there, fight and resist the gravity of the weight, lowering the stack as slowly as possible. Perform two or three negative reps in this style. This procedure maximizes stress on the muscles that control the negative part of the rep and leads to optimum size and strength gains.

WEIDER DESCENDING SETS TRAINING PRINCIPLE

The descending sets principle is similar to forced reps except that you don't necessarily need a partner to use it. Descending sets are best used for exercises that allow quick transitions from your working weight to a lower weight. Exercises that require dumbbells or a machine with a stack of weights are ideal. For instance, utilizing the descending sets principle is quite effective with triceps pressdowns. Perform your regular set until you reach failure. Quickly move the pin on the stack, reducing the weight by 20-30%. With this lighter poundage, perform as many reps as possible with absolute strict form, stopping when you reach form break for the second time.

to complete a series of partial reps. Partial reps are particularly effective for exercises that don't lend themselves well to the forced reps, rest-pause or negative reps principles, such as lateral raises or leg extensions.

Using leg extensions as an example, here's how the Weider Partial Reps Training Principle works. Once you hit failure, continue to raise your lower legs as high as possible, without shuffling around on the seat or using any other form of cheating. You may be able to do two or three three-quarter-range reps in this style. As you tire, the movement will decrease to half reps; do two or three in this range. Finally, do two or three reps of a quarter-range movement to finish the set.

For partials to be effective, it's imperative that you continue to use perfect form through the phase of the rep that you are still performing. Don't allow yourself cheating motions such as bouncing off the seat. Instead, keep the attention wholly focused on your quads, and continue to work them as hard as you can. Although you won't be able to get a full contraction, you're still working them harder than if you had stopped after your last full rep.

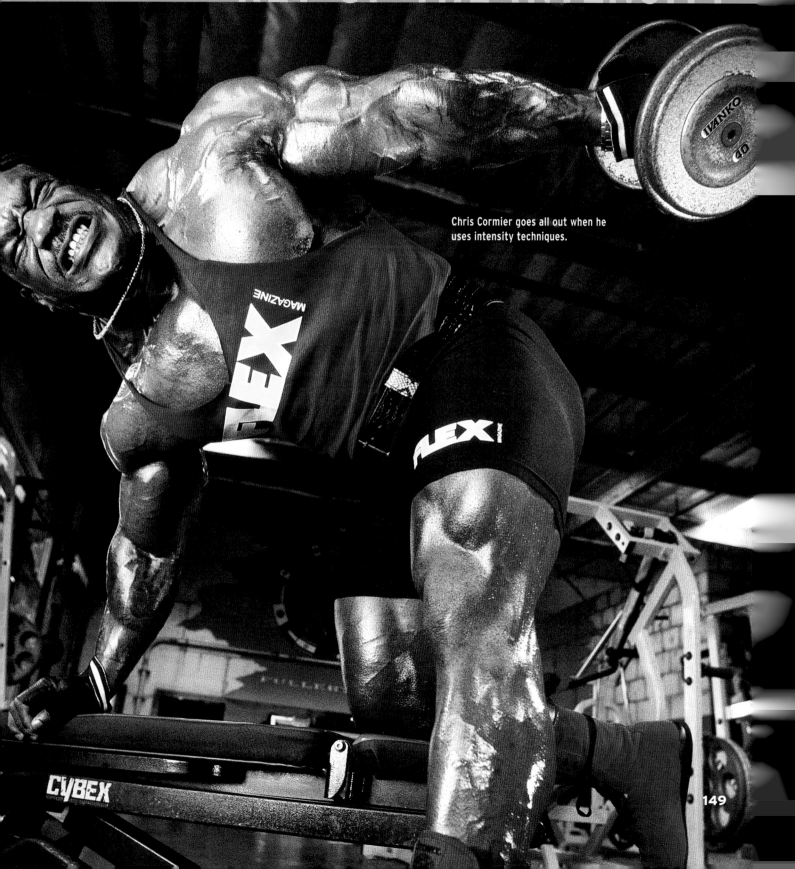

Chris Cormier goes all out when he uses intensity techniques.

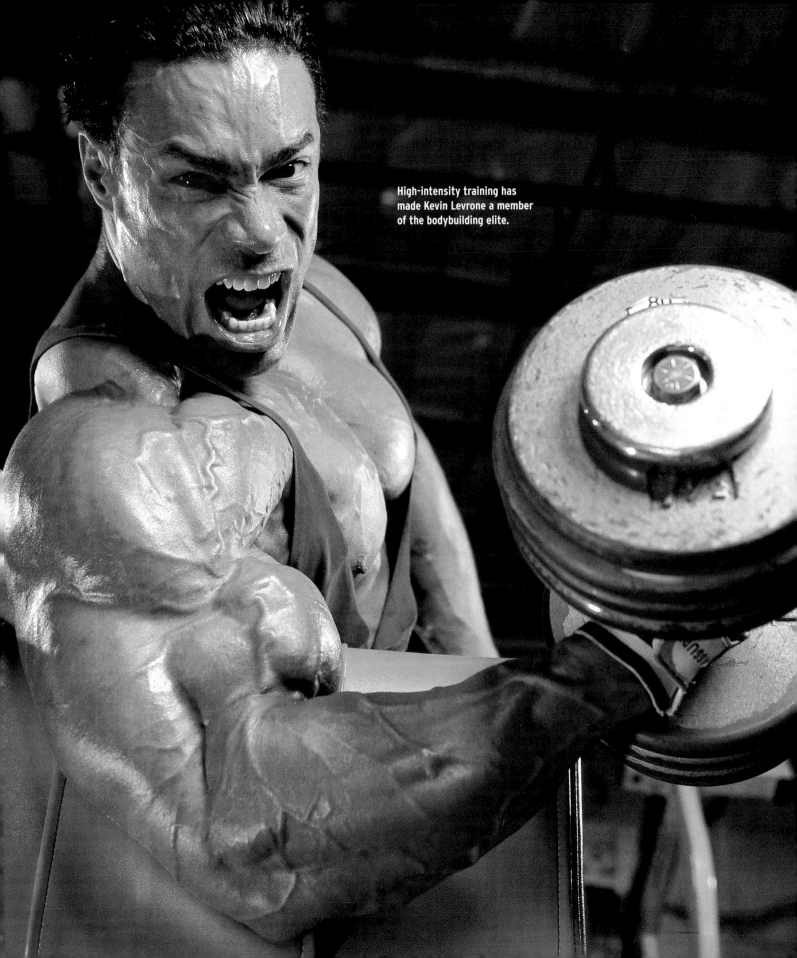

High-intensity training has made Kevin Levrone a member of the bodybuilding elite.

Shock THERAPY

Shake up an ordinary training routine with these shock tactics

Bodybuilding has long had an unusual appeal. You were probably first attracted to the sport by images of massive muscles and the question "How does a person get to look like that?" The first trip to a well-equipped gym is often perplexing. With training experience, however, bodybuilding can become as familiar as brushing your teeth. Although today's top bodybuilders can make anyone's jaw drop, there's probably nothing shocking about your current workout program. That's when familiarity starts working against you.

You need to rekindle the feeling you had when bodybuilding was fresh and exciting for you, when utilizing certain exercises or techniques made you sore — and made you grow. You need to make every workout an adventure, just like it used to be. This may require a rededication to your present program and goals, or a completely different style of training.

The following methodologies are not generally intended to replace your current training program. They shock your muscles to new growth in one to three weeks. Then, you can return to your usual program with new intensity and enthusiasm. Keep an open mind, but don't abandon any routine if it's safe, effective and you're happy with it. Don't follow any of these recommendations for longer than a month.

THE CIRCUIT

Circuit training is a form of aerobic exercise in which one set for a bodypart is followed quickly by another set for a

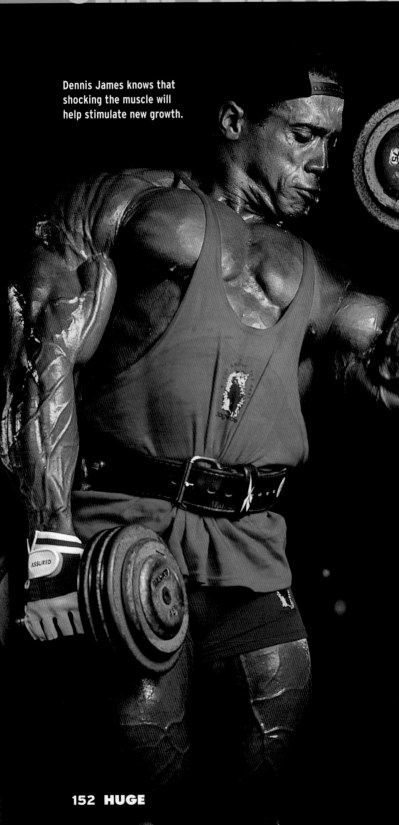

Dennis James knows that shocking the muscle will help stimulate new growth.

different bodypart until you've done one exercise for every muscle group. Three to five such circuits are typically performed per workout.

One circuit might consist of squats, bench presses, lat pulldowns, leg curls, crunches, shoulder presses, calf raises, triceps extensions and biceps curls — in that order. If you're pressed for time and can line up nine separate workout stations, circuit training allows you to work your entire body in a half-hour. It can also give you an effective cardio boost. Circuit training is certainly a unique method of weight training. Although it's good for an occasional shock, it doesn't let you work your muscles long and hard enough to make them grow. Trisets and giant sets for unrelated bodyparts can be a form of circuit training. For example, you might want to try a powerlifting triset, going from squats to bench presses to deadlifts with virtually no rest. Do three to five such trisets, keeping the reps above 10. Rest one minute or less between circuits.

You can do triset or giant-set circuits using numerous exercise combinations — for instance, pulldowns to shoulder presses to triceps pushdowns to biceps curls. Most weight-training exercises can be used in circuit training, but do only one exercise per bodypart. Most important, don't rest during the circuit, and rest very little between circuits.

You might want to circuit train on a day other than a regular workout day, perhaps when you work abs, calves or do aerobics. If you're burned out on your normal routine, do only circuits every other day for a few weeks.

HIGH SETS

The workouts of today's top pros generally aren't as long as those of past champions. For instance, in his heyday, three-time Mr. Olympia Sergio Oliva pumped away for hours each session. Robby Robinson, 1977 and 1978 Mr. Olympia runner-up, did as many as 50 sets for thighs and 32 sets for calves per workout. Roy Callender, 1977 IFBB Universe middleweight winner, did more than 80 sets for lats per session, including 28 sets of weighted chins. Callender was a firm believer in a full workday. Before a contest, he trained for eight out of every 24 hours!

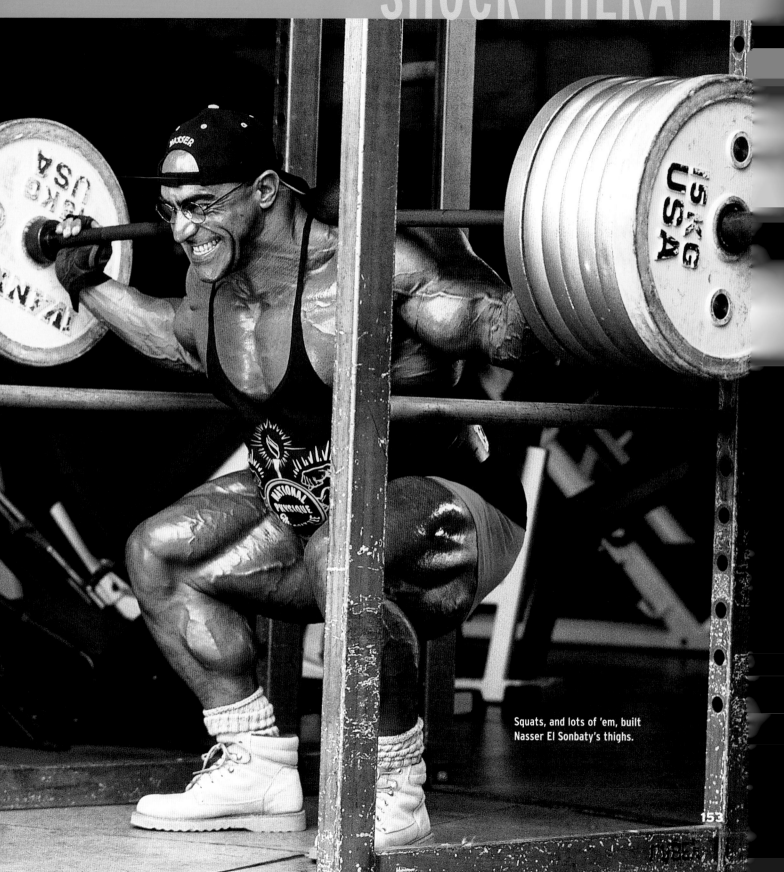

SHOCK THERAPY

Squats, and lots of 'em, built
Nasser El Sonbaty's thighs.

One way to increase stress on muscle is to raise the volume of work. This principle probably worked well during your first year of training as you went from beginner to intermediate. However, hiking the volume has its limitations. Performing more than 20 sets per bodypart in one workout can lead to overtraining. This rule doesn't hold true for everyone, though, as seen with Oliva, Robinson and Callender. Like most muscle-building rules, you can break this one for a while to shock your muscles.

If you increase from 15 sets to 25 while working chest, attempting the same intensity, your pecs will be sore — and will grow. However, they'll require more time to recover. Boosting workout volume from 50% to 100% by adding two or three more exercises is an excellent way to shock complacent

For high intensity, you must hate to put the weight down. Always struggle to keep a set going and your muscles working.

muscles, but without adequate rest, it can lead to overtraining. You need at least one additional recuperation day before training a volume-overloaded bodypart again.

An alternate high-volume method is to focus on only one exercise per workout. For example, Arnold Schwarzenegger fondly remembers training sessions in his youth in which he did countless sets of squats until he could barely stand. If you make one exercise the focus of a workout (20 or more sets), it should be a basic compound exercise such as deadlifts, squats, leg presses, bench presses or power cleans.

During a regular workout, you can also do one exercise per bodypart instead of three or four. Keep your total sets per bodypart the same. For example, instead of performing four sets each of preacher curls, dumbbell curls and cable curls, do 12 sets of barbell curls. The repetition overload of doing only one exercise when a muscle is accustomed to various exercises should force that muscle to grow.

MEGA-HIGH REPS
Like circuit training, very high repetitions are generally associated with aerobics and light conditioning exercises.

However, when used sparingly, reps in the 30-100 range can shock your muscles. Mega-high reps often provide two growth bursts — one while performing high reps for a few weeks and the other after resuming your regular workouts.

A great way to shock your thighs is to stay away from the gym and do one super-high-rep set of nonstop deep knee bends, touching glutes to ankles during each rep. If you think this sounds easy, you'll probably change your mind after doing more than 500 without stopping. You can achieve the same effect with weight-free lunges.

HIGH INTENSITY
Another way to shock your muscles is to increase workout intensity. The following Weider Training Principles can help you boost intensity beyond the norm: supersets, descending sets, negative reps, forced reps, rest-pause, cheating, partial reps and burns, continuous tension, iso-tension and peak contraction. Each of these principles can shock your muscles the first few times used. (See the previous chapter for more information on the Weider Training Principles.) If you already employ them in your training, the best way to shock your muscles is to combine several principles and maximize your mental intensity.

As strenuous as the previous example might seem, it doesn't do justice to what high intensity really is. You must hate to put the weight down. Always struggle to keep a set going and your muscles working. High-intensity training is a way of life for many top bodybuilders, but in short bursts, it can also blast muscle toward new growth, returning power and purpose to your effort. Even more important than with the previous techniques, warm up properly and use spotters when pushing beyond your normal limits.

SHOCK ABSORBING
Despite the "shocking" language used here, don't just jump in and jar or injure your muscles with this shock therapy. Take at least a week to ease into it. Carefully increase your reps, sets and intensity from one workout to the next.

Say no to complacency and ordinary routines. Travel back to the time when weight training was new and exciting for you. Armed with the courage to try something different, you can break out of a training slump and force your muscles to grow, just as you did the first time you picked up a weight — back when everything was shocking.

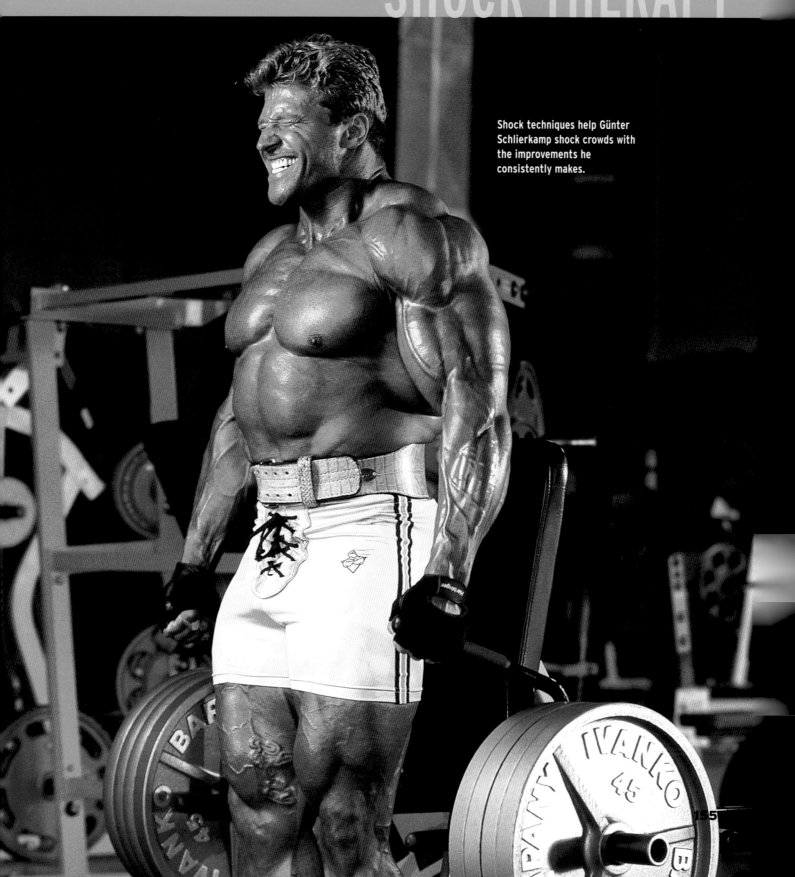

Shock techniques help Günter Schlierkamp shock crowds with the improvements he consistently makes.

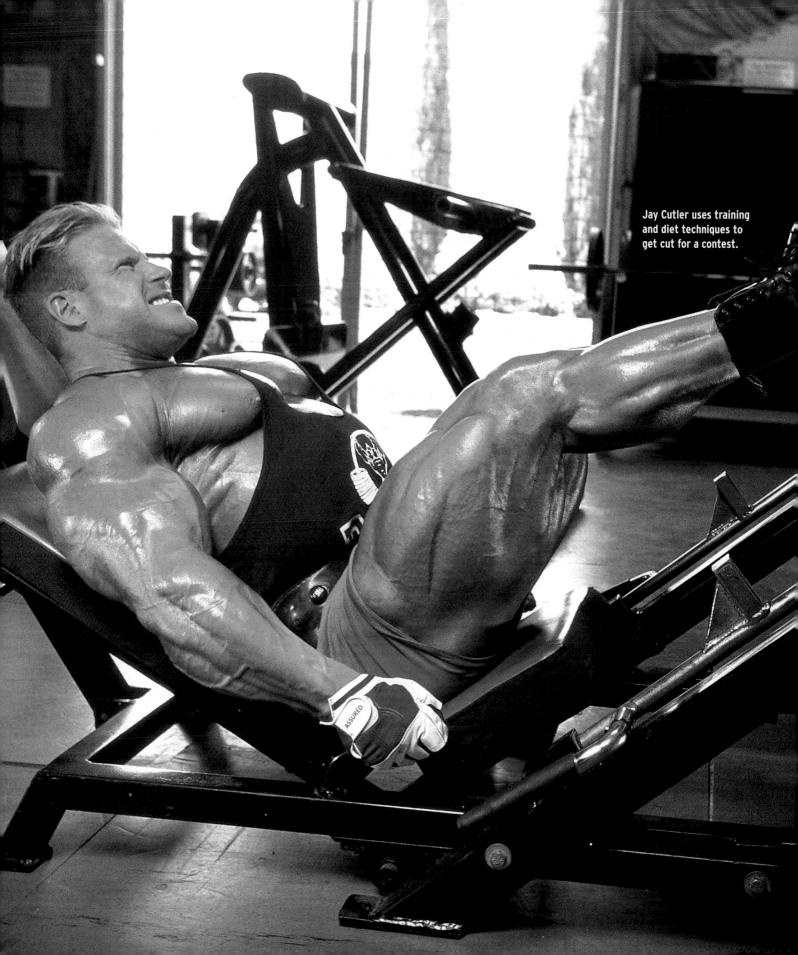

Jay Cutler uses training and diet techniques to get cut for a contest.

RIP IT UP

This program will get you cut while maintaining muscle mass

IMPORTANT NOTE

If you want to continue building size rather than go into a cutting-up phase, you should, instead of following the regimen outlined in this chapter, refer to the 13-week Power Surge segment in Chapter 10. Adhering to the Power Surge program will keep your mass-building momentum going, and you can pick up the cutting-up phase at a later date.

Bodybuilding is a sport about size and the illusion of size. At no time are these potentially conflicting goals more in sync than in a cutting phase of training. During this process, you're trying to maintain the muscle you've acquired as you reduce your bodyfat, creating the appearance of carrying even more muscle mass. This is accomplished by keeping as much fullness in your upper body and legs as possible while reducing the size of your midsection. It's inevitable that some size will come off your legs and upper body as you diet off bodyfat, but the differential in tightening your midsection helps create the appearance of having greater overall size and muscularity. To reduce bodyfat while maintaining muscle mass, you need a specific protocol and you must follow it rigidly to get the best results.

We've broken down this phase into three major components: weight training, cardiovascular training and nutrition. In this chapter we describe a 13-week weight training and cardio program. In pursuit of cutting up, you need to burn more calories than normal, and nothing aids that process like a regular cardio regimen. For the nutrition plan, see Chapter 17.

The focus of this cutting-up phase is to produce a full and ripped physique at the end of 13 weeks. Don't diet strictly in the first month. The shock of suddenly training differently and doing regular cardio is sufficient for now. At this point, simply clean up your eating habits.

SECTION ONE: WEIGHT TRAINING

As you enter this final phase, you've already built the muscle; now it's time to concentrate on the presentation. One truism of bodybuilding is that it's much easier to maintain muscle mass than it is to acquire it. Previously, you've been training individual bodyparts in a strategy designed to add as much muscle as possible. Now, you want to hold onto that size as you reduce bodyfat, and that calls for a different weight-training protocol.

In this training regimen, you will use mainly compound exercises (often called basic exercises), which are the prime movements for building mass. Compound exercises concentrate on major muscle groups, but also call into play auxiliary muscles. For instance, bench presses focus mainly on the chest muscles, but recruit the delts and triceps as auxiliaries. This allows you to handle much heavier poundages than would be the case in chest isolation exercises such as flyes, which do not recruit secondary muscle groups. Compound movements allow you to handle the heaviest weights for each bodypart. They are, therefore, the prime

exercises for maintaining mass. The exception to the compound rule is abs — high-rep sets will burn fat from and

In this training regimen, you will use mainly compound exercises, which are the prime movements for building mass.

sculpt the midsection.

For the first month, divide your weight training into four weekly sessions — two upper body, two lower body. On Mondays and Thursdays, train chest, back, shoulders, biceps, triceps and abs. Apart from abs, do one exercise each for five sets of six reps. Choose the heaviest weight that allows you to complete this amount. During the first four sets, you may be

WEIGHT WORKOUT

EXERCISE	BODYPART	WEEKS 1-4		WEEKS 5-13	
		SETS	REPS	SETS	REPS
MONDAY					
Bench presses	Chest	5	6	5	10
Barbell rows	Back	5	6	5	10
Dumbbell presses	Shoulders	5	6	5	10
Seated dumbbell curls	Biceps	5	6	5	10
Rope pressdowns	Triceps	5	6	5	10
Crunches	Abs	5	20	5	20
TUESDAY					
Leg curls	Hamstrings	5	6	5	10
Squats	Quads	5	6	5	10
Good mornings	Lower back	5	6	5	10
Smith machine squats	Quads	5	6	5	10
Donkey calf raises	Calves	5	6	5	10
THURSDAY					
Incline bench presses	Chest	5	6	5	10
Chinups	Back	5	6	5	10
Seated barbell presses	Shoulders	5	6	5	10
90-degree preacher curls	Biceps	5	6	5	10
Seated triceps extensions	Triceps	5	6	5	10
Reverse crunches	Abs	5	20	5	20
FRIDAY					
Deadlifts	Back	5	6	5	10
Leg presses	Quads	5	6	5	10
Leg curls	Hamstrings	5	6	5	10
Hyperextensions	Lower back	5	6	5	10
Seated calf raises	Calves	5	6	5	10

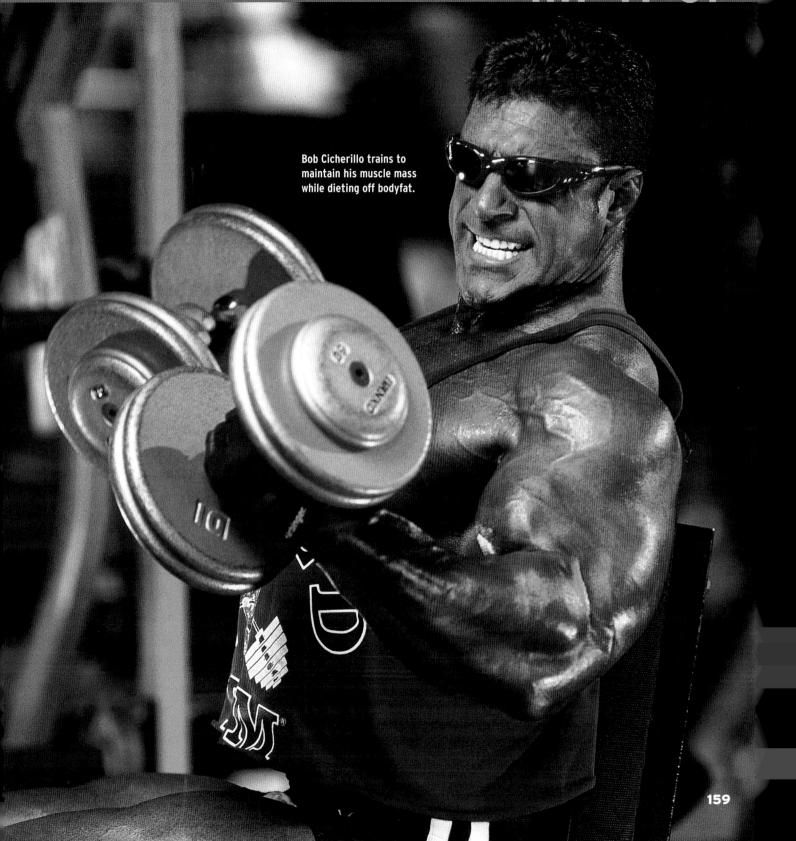

Bob Cicherillo trains to maintain his muscle mass while dieting off bodyfat.

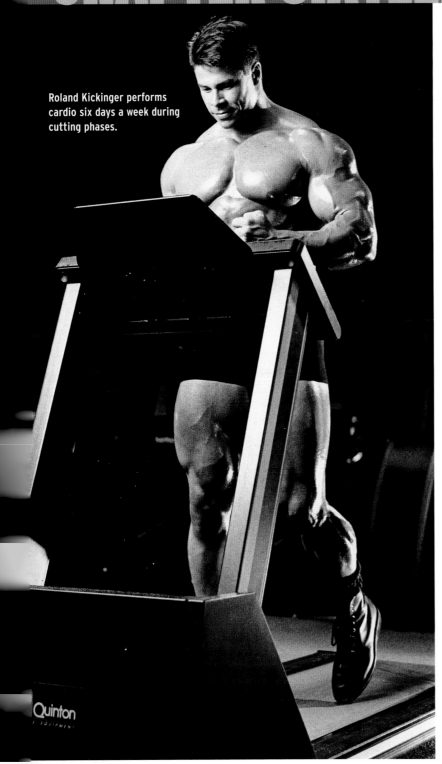

Roland Kickinger performs cardio six days a week during cutting phases.

able to pump out more, but stop at six reps for each set. Rest periods should be neither too short nor too long — rest long enough to feel recovered from the previous set and ready to perform the next. Keep in mind that you're not trying to take your muscles to failure on every set — you're trying to provide them with the appropriate stimulation for maintenance.

On Tuesdays and Fridays, you'll primarily train your lower body. The exercises used target either the entire lower body (such as deadlifts and Smith machine squats), or specific bodyparts (leg curls for hamstrings, donkey calf raises for calves).

Use the 5x6 set-and-rep scheme for weeks one through four on all weight-training workouts, and then switch to a 5x10 set-and-rep scheme for weeks five through 13. As with the first four weeks, choose a weight that allows you complete the fifth set of 10 reps. Stop at 10 reps in the first four sets even if you can perform more reps with that weight. Increasing reps to 10 during the second month is an important part of the overall cutting phase. Higher reps will provide your body with more of a pump, burn more calories and allow you to add more detail to your musculature.

SECTION TWO: CARDIOVASCULAR TRAINING

Cardiovascular training is a crucial component of burning bodyfat. So, it would seem to make sense that the more cardio you perform, the more bodyfat you burn. But that's not necessarily true — the human body is far more complicated than that. To get the most out of your cardiovascular training, you need to be aware of how your body responds to cardiovascular work so that you can train appropriately in terms of duration, intensity and time of day.

The type of cardio you choose can vary. Most bodybuilders walk on a slightly inclined treadmill because that provides a steady workload where you move your entire bodyweight, reducing the potential of overuse and impact injuries. Other cardio options, including outdoor walking, slow jogging, stationary cycling or stair climbing, can be equally effective. Feel free to mix and match cardiovascular options to make life more interesting.

Whichever you choose, you don't need to work at high intensity at all times. Surprisingly, pushing yourself beyond 75% effort can burn less bodyfat than working at a lower effort level. The harder you work, the more you tend to burn carbs you've recently consumed. Although you might burn more overall calories, you might also end up burning fewer calories from stored bodyfat. Working at 50-70% intensity is a better strategy, as you'll burn a greater amount of calories from stored bodyfat and still leave yourself with enough muscle glycogen to handle heavy weights. A purposeful walking pace (three or four miles per hour) on a three- to seven-degree inclined treadmill approximates this range for most trained individuals.

CARDIO WORKOUT

DAY	WEEKS 1-13 DURATION*	INTENSITY	TIMING
MONDAY	30 minutes	50-60%	Posttraining
TUESDAY	30 minutes	50-60%	Posttraining
WEDNESDAY (optional)	60 minutes	60-70% max	Morning
THURSDAY	30 minutes	50-60%	Posttraining
FRIDAY	30 minutes	50-60%	Posttraining
SATURDAY (optional)	60 minutes	60-70% max	Morning
SUNDAY	Rest		

*If you feel up to it, add five minutes every second week to all posttraining cardio sessions.

We advocate that you do 30 minutes of cardio following each of your workouts.

The duration and timing of your cardiovascular training vary based on your weightlifting. We advocate that you do 30 minutes of cardio following each of your workouts. However, if you start to lose significant muscle mass, cut back on the cardio and experiment with the amount of sessions that enable you to retain your hard-won muscle. On the other hand, if your fitness level permits and you really want to crank it up, try an extra hour of cardio on Wednesdays and Saturdays, or just on one of those days.

On Wednesdays and Saturdays, days when you don't weight train, the optimal time for cardio sessions is first thing in the morning on an empty stomach. After you consume food, your blood sugar rises, and your body will preferentially utilize that source for energy. When you start exercising after a lengthy period of inactivity, it takes your body awhile — usually about 15 minutes — to make the adaptations necessary to tap into bodyfat. Therefore, make these your long cardiovascular sessions of the week. An hour is ideal, and exercising at 60-70% effort helps maximize fat burning.

On days when you weight train, FLEX recommends that you complete both weight and cardio workouts in one stop at the gym if possible. After weight training, consume a postworkout meal, then wait 20 minutes or so before hitting the cardio. After exercising, you have increased blood flow, and your body will be able to tap into bodyfat stores in these relatively short cardio sessions. Taking in your postworkout meal beforehand helps provide the necessary nutrients for rebuilding muscle mass after weight training, but also provides some calories to burn during cardio. If you have enough energy left after weight training, you can opt to postpone your postworkout shake until after your cardio to enhance burning bodyfat.

SECTION THREE: NUTRITION

At this point, nutrition is a concern, but only a secondary one. Focus on cleaning up your diet and preparing your body for the much more rigorous nutrition plan outlined in the next chapter. To clean up your diet, begin implementing the following rules.

- Eat whole foods. This is the single biggest shift you should make in your diet over the first month of this phase. Try to construct as much of your diet as possible from simply prepared meats, vegetables, fruits, whole eggs, nuts and whole grains. In general, the more similar a food is to the way it appears in nature, the more appropriate it is to a bodybuilding cutting phase.
- Reduce consumption of white flour as much as possible.

Refined flour is one of the worst foods for bodybuilders, and especially for those trying to shed bodyfat. Eliminate crackers, snack foods, white bread (and buns) and

important to eat a nutritious meal or have a protein shake as soon as you feel hungry.

■ Allow yourself a cheat food or two a week. Cutting phases

In general, the more similar a food is to the way it appears in nature, the more appropriate it is to a bodybuilding cutting phase.

even pastas made from white flour. Replace them with whole-grain substitutes, but try to reduce overall consumption of these starches as much as you can. To keep your calories in balance, use brown rice, oatmeal, yams and other complex carbs. They're slower burning than other starches and won't affect your blood sugar as much, ultimately priming your body to tap into fat stores more effectively.

■ Reduce consumption of sugar. Cut out sodas, fruit juices and other sugary drinks. Other sources of sugar, including desserts, candy and milk, should also be cut. The only exception is to continue to take in your postworkout drink of 50-100 grams of simple carbs and 30-50 grams of protein. At this stage, keep your glycogen stores full so that you have all the muscular energy you need for weight training and cardio.

■ Drink as much water as possible and supplement with vitamins and minerals. Be particularly vigilant about hydration and mineral supplementation. With the increase in cardio, you will excrete more water and minerals than you have in previous phases. In general, consume at least a gallon of water a day (in addition to water from other sources), and follow FLEX's recommendations for vitamin and mineral supplementation in Chapter 7.

■ Don't focus on cutting calories. If you reduce your calories too much too quickly, you'll drop more weight than you want to — much of it hard-earned muscle. During this first month, in fact, you should put effort into increasing your food volume. Since, overall, the foods you are eating should have fewer calories, you need to eat more to get the same calories. Keep in mind that you are also increasing your energy expenditure by increasing cardio training, so the overall effect on your body will be a calorie deficit. As a rule of thumb, at no time should you be hungry during this month. Hunger is a warning that you are burning off muscle mass, so it's

work better if you give yourself a little slack rather than if you instantly launch into a different style of eating. Once or twice a week, treat yourself to a cheat food, but in moderation. Have a small burger instead of a super-sized fast-food extravaganza. Share a dessert instead of eating one by yourself.

■ Read labels. If a food has a long list of chemicals that you don't recognize, you can be sure it's not a whole food. Leave it on the grocery shelf and head for the produce section or meat counter.

NOW CUT TO THE CHASE

Follow the guidelines prescribed in this chapter and you will be on the path to shaping a ripped and full physique. In the next chapter, we'll increase the fat-burning intensity with a formal cutting-up diet. Until then, keep lifting those weights and doing that cardio.

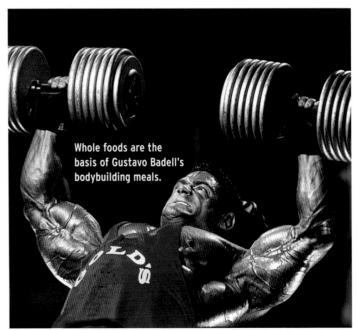

Whole foods are the basis of Gustavo Badell's bodybuilding meals.

During cutting phases, Troy Alves eschews processed foods.

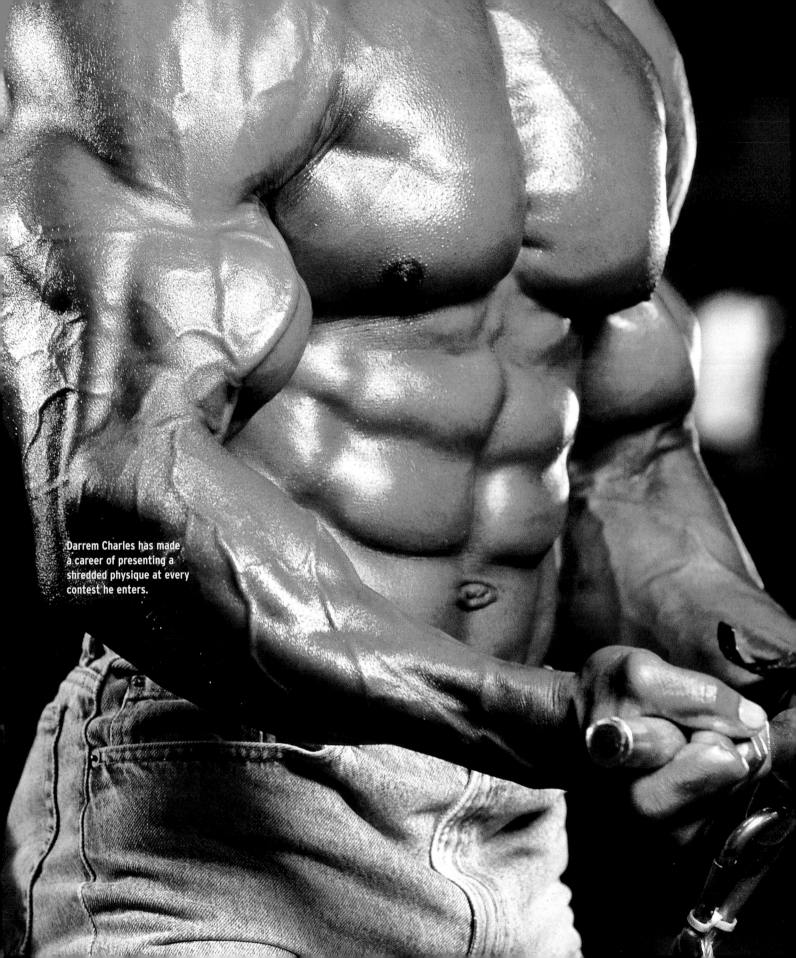

Darrem Charles has made a career of presenting a shredded physique at every contest he enters.

SHREDDED

This eight-week nutrition program will get you more ripped than you've ever been

In the last chapter, we introduced the "Rip It Up" training regimen, a 13-week cutting-up workout designed to get you started on reducing bodyfat while retaining muscle mass and as an initial step toward cleaning up your diet. In this chapter, we'll help you take it up a notch with an eight-week nutrition program.

The prep work is as important as the diet itself: It takes time for your body to process the message that you want to pull fat from storage and to make the necessary accommodations. Now you're ready to begin the diet phase of this program. On this nutrition regimen, you will reduce bodyfat using the following three diet strategies.

1. Rev up your metabolic rate by providing your body with several meals a day. It's important to add at least one more meal than you were previously eating to help your body increase its metabolic rate. Ideally, you should eat six or more meals a day.

2. Reduce calories from carbohydrates and increase calories from protein. Eating too many carbohydrate calories reduces the body's ability to burn fat.

3. Reduce calorie-dense foods, but maintain nearly the same daily caloric intake. When you reduce complex carbs and replace them with vegetables and replace fatty protein

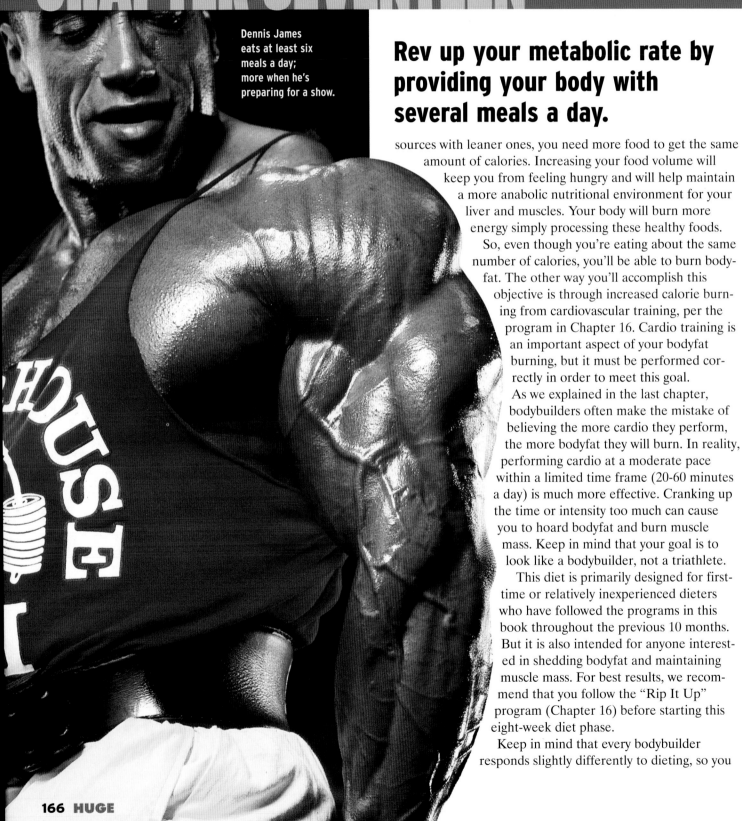

Dennis James eats at least six meals a day; more when he's preparing for a show.

Rev up your metabolic rate by providing your body with several meals a day.

sources with leaner ones, you need more food to get the same amount of calories. Increasing your food volume will keep you from feeling hungry and will help maintain a more anabolic nutritional environment for your liver and muscles. Your body will burn more energy simply processing these healthy foods.

So, even though you're eating about the same number of calories, you'll be able to burn body-fat. The other way you'll accomplish this objective is through increased calorie burning from cardiovascular training, per the program in Chapter 16. Cardio training is an important aspect of your bodyfat burning, but it must be performed correctly in order to meet this goal.

As we explained in the last chapter, bodybuilders often make the mistake of believing the more cardio they perform, the more bodyfat they will burn. In reality, performing cardio at a moderate pace within a limited time frame (20-60 minutes a day) is much more effective. Cranking up the time or intensity too much can cause you to hoard bodyfat and burn muscle mass. Keep in mind that your goal is to look like a bodybuilder, not a triathlete.

This diet is primarily designed for first-time or relatively inexperienced dieters who have followed the programs in this book throughout the previous 10 months. But it is also intended for anyone interested in shedding bodyfat and maintaining muscle mass. For best results, we recommend that you follow the "Rip It Up" program (Chapter 16) before starting this eight-week diet phase.

Keep in mind that every bodybuilder responds slightly differently to dieting, so you

SHREDDED

might have to make adjustments for your specific needs (see "Diet Harder" on page 183). As a guide to meal planning, we offer an example (see "Diet Hard Meal Plan" on page 180). The following discussion gives you all the information you need to design the ideal diet plan for your individual needs.

KNOW YOUR NUTRIENTS
As you put your meal plan together, you need to focus on the following nutrients and foods.

PROTEIN Protein consumption is as important during a cutting phase as it is in a growth phase. During a growth phase, you need protein to help you gain more muscle mass. During a cutting phase, you need protein to help you maintain the

six meals a day, split your complex carbs as follows: meals one and three: 50-75 g; meals two and four: 50 g or fewer; meals five and six: no measurable carbs. Complex carbs eaten late at night tend to be stored as bodyfat because they are not immediately utilized for energy.

Ideal sources of complex carbs include sweet potatoes, oatmeal and brown rice, which are slow-burning and provide you with a better sense of satiety and energy per calorie than other complex carbs do. Other good sources include baked potatoes, white rice and whole-grain bread, but try to emphasize the first group over the second.

HEALTHY FATS To reduce bodyfat, remove unhealthy saturated and trans fats from your nutrition plan, but don't eliminate

Strive to take in at least 30 grams of protein at each meal, including shakes and whole foods such as meat, fish and eggs.

muscle mass you've already acquired and to provide a source of energy when carb intake is reduced. It's very easy to lose muscle mass as you diet. Muscle is one of the most readily available energy sources, and your body will preferentially burn it off unless you provide an alternative.

Take in at least one gram (g) of protein per pound of bodyweight each day. Protein should be spread fairly evenly throughout the day. Strive to take in at least 30 g of protein at each meal, including shakes and whole foods such as meat, fish and eggs. Because of the overall reduction in other nutrients, you might need to increase protein consumption to maintain muscle mass while you burn bodyfat. In fact, bumping protein intake up to 1.25-1.5 g per pound of bodyweight per day will definitely help you retain mass and strength as you lean out.

COMPLEX CARBS To reduce bodyfat, you need to consume fewer carbs each day. Complex carbs provide energy and fuel, and they help you put on size — in the forms of both muscle and bodyfat. During a cutting phase, it's reasonable to take in 1-1.5 g of complex carbs per pound of bodyweight each day. (You shouldn't be eating simple carbs other than those in postworkout drinks, plus small amounts of fruit.)

If you weigh 200 pounds, you can take in 200-300 g of carbs. Consume them early in the day. For instance, if you eat

fats altogether. Even though you're in a cutting phase, 10-15% of your calories should come from healthy fats. These fats are particularly helpful in a cutting phase as they provide a sense of satiety and may also drastically reduce cravings for simple carbs.

Excellent sources of healthy fats include avocados, flaxseed and olive oils, fatty fish such as salmon, and all-natural peanut butter. A spoonful of peanut butter makes a great snack and also seems to reduce cravings for carbs for many

DIET HARD CHECKLIST
Keep this handy list of reminders with you.
- Drink water, water, water
- Eat fiber: fruits, vegetables, fiber supplements and oatmeal
- Eat starchy carbs in the morning and right after training
- At night, no carbs except vegetables and fiber
- Drink a postworkout shake of protein and simple carbs
- Drink a midafternoon protein shake that includes carbs
- Supplement with creatine to help keep muscles full
- Supplement with glutamine to aid in recovery
- Supplement with flaxseed oil for satiety, health and well-being
- Take a daily multivitamin/multimineral to ensure you have no deficiencies
- Eat six or more meals a day

bodybuilders. Watch the quantity, though, and buy brands that contain no added sugar and not much salt. Remember that these foods are calorically dense, and eating a large quantity will take you beyond your calorie threshold for losing bodyfat.

VEGETABLES For first-time dieters in particular, steamed vegetables are essentially a "free" food — you can eat as much of them as you want. Often, dieters count them toward their carbohydrate limits, but, as long as you avoid large quantities of starchy vegetables such as peas, carrots and corn, you can eat an unlimited amount. The calories contained in cauliflower, broccoli, zucchini and spinach and other leafy vegetables are minimal compared to their advantages. These vegetables provide your body with a great deal of food volume, which helps you feel satiated and keeps you from eating foods you should avoid. Food volume also

During a cutting phase, you need protein to help you maintain the muscle mass you've already acquired.

assists your digestive process. Consuming vegetables with protein makes it easier to digest and absorb, and this makes your overall diet more efficient.

In addition, vegetables are loaded with nutrients and fiber. The vitamins and minerals they contain will help ensure that you have no deficiencies in your diet as you reduce bodyfat. Fiber — one of the most overlooked aspects of bodybuilding nutrition — in vegetables helps scrub the colon and is instrumental in providing food volume.

FRUITS Fruits also contain fiber, helping to increase food volume. In addition, they offer a bundle of vitamins and other beneficial phytochemicals. Fruit is a key part of a healthy bodybuilding diet, but you should not rely too heavily on fruit while you are trying to reduce bodyfat. A piece or two a day is fine.

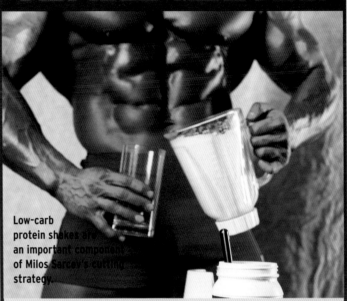

DIET HARD MEAL PLAN

Low-carb protein shakes are an important component of Milos Sarcev's cutting strategy.

This sample meal plan is for one day only and provides you with an example of how you might construct your diet program. Each day, substitute different foods to make sure you're providing your body with a variety of nutrients.

Strive to take in nearly the same number of calories you were consuming before you began the diet — if you fall 100-200 calories short, that's OK, as long as you aren't losing muscle mass in the process. Make adjustments in the quantity of protein and fats you consume if you need to add more calories to your diet.

MEAL ONE: 7 AM
6 egg whites
50-75 g oatmeal
4 slices fat-free turkey bacon

MEAL TWO: 10 AM
Midmorning protein shake (no carbs)

MEAL THREE: 12 noon
Turkey sandwich (one slice of bread piled high with meat, plus a few slices of avocado and olive for taste)
Salad with fat-free dressing or healthy oil-based dressing

MEAL FOUR: 2:30 PM
Midafternoon protein shake of 30-50 g protein and 30 g carbs
Small sweet potato or baked potato

WORKOUT: 5 PM

MEAL FIVE: 6:30 PM
Postworkout shake — at least 30 g protein, 30-50 g carbs, followed a half-hour later by 8 oz chicken, fish or lean red meat
Large helping of steamed vegetables (or salad)

MEAL SIX: 9 PM
Protein shake (no carbs)
2 tablespoons peanut butter

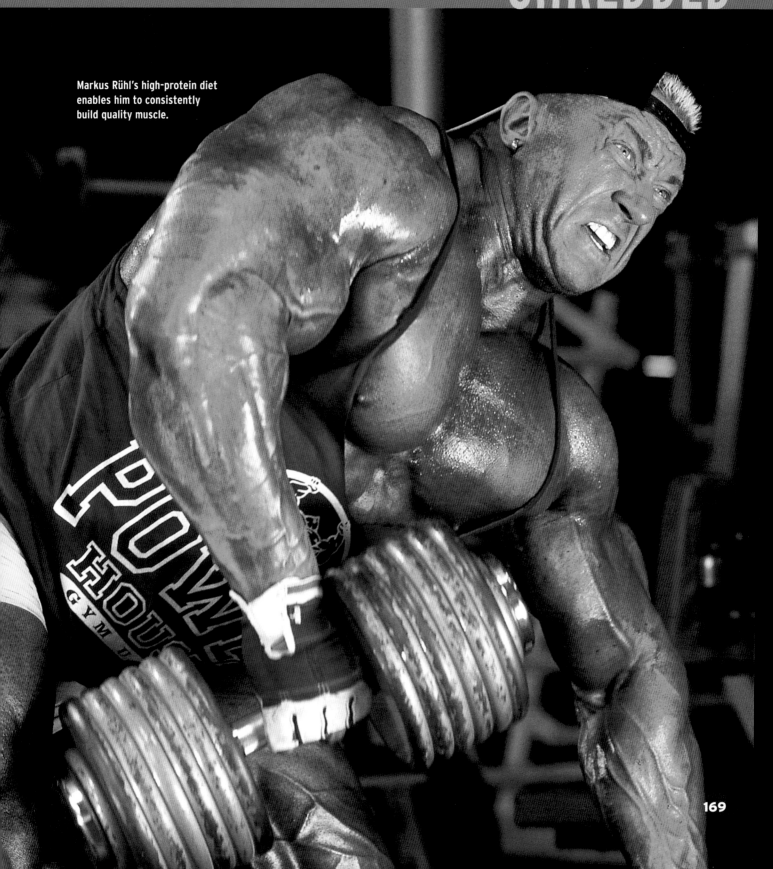

Markus Rühl's high-protein diet enables him to consistently build quality muscle.

To present a pumped and ripped physique, Kevin Levrone carefully monitored his contest diet.

DIET HARDER
Make these adjustments if you're losing weight too slowly or too quickly

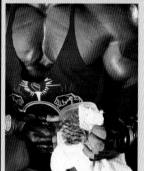

After following the diet for two to three weeks, make an honest evaluation of your progress. The first week of dieting will normally produce a greater loss of weight than subsequent weeks, because you tend to reduce water weight when you cut carbohydrates. Having added cardiovascular training and cleaned up your diet in the previous month, though, should prevent you from dumping too much weight too quickly.

Your body can pull only so much bodyfat from storage during a week. You shouldn't expect to lose more than two pounds of bodyfat weekly, for a highly optimistic six to eight pounds of bodyfat a month. If you're losing more than that, you're shedding muscle mass. If you're losing significantly less than that, you should make some adjustments. Here are some recommendations to help your diet work better.

TO LOSE MORE BODYFAT
- Increase the amount of time devoted to cardio. Perform 30-minute sessions after each weight workout and add one or two hourlong cardio sessions on nontraining days. During 30-minute sessions, cycle the intensity. Work at a moderate pace for a few minutes, then crank up the intensity (to 90%) for 30 seconds. Cut back to a lesser intensity, say 50-60% for 60-90 seconds, then push the intensity again. Do this for 20-25 minutes.
- Cut complex carbs to a total of 150 g per day. You may need to restrict calories a little more than other people to get the desired results. Don't reduce complex carbs drastically or cut calories below 1,800. If you do, you'll send your body the message that it's enduring a period of near-starvation, which will make it want to hoard bodyfat.

TO SLOW DOWN WEIGHT LOSS
- Bump up complex carbs to a total of 250 g per day. Add these carbs to meals at which you're already consuming complex carbs. Don't add them to late-night meals.
- Perform 30 minutes of easy cardio after each weight workout — consider walking on a flat treadmill over other options. Drop the extra hourlong sessions and skip the intense intervals. If your body burns calories like crazy when you do cardio, you might have to reduce the time and intensity to keep from burning off your newly acquired muscle mass.
- Eat more protein and vegetables at each meal. You might not be taking in enough total calories. Chicken breasts and vegetables are not as calorically dense as the food you're accustomed to eating, yet you might be consuming the same food volume as before. Boost the volume to compensate for the lower caloric density.
- Allow two cheat foods per week. You might be restricting your calories too much, especially considering the increased energy demands you're making on your body.

You should try to consume at least a gallon of water a day in addition to other beverages.

WATER Like fiber, water is another overlooked aspect of bodybuilding nutrition. Regardless of the phase of your bodybuilding, you should try to consume at least a gallon of water a day in addition to other beverages. When you diet, it's even more critical. Water helps hydrate your body and flush toxins from your system. It also provides you with nutrients via its mineral content. Drink water throughout the day, especially between meals and before, during and after your workout.

CHEAT FOODS If you have the discipline to avoid cheat foods, great. Avoid them. If you don't, make accommodations for them in your diet. Allow yourself 100-200 calories or so of a favorite cheat food once or twice a week. Plan out those cheat sessions, adhere to your schedule and reward yourself for making it three or four days without a cookie or a small slice of pizza. But keep cheating to an absolute minimum. There's simply no point in enduring many days of deprivation only to sabotage it with a bingefest that undoes all your hard work.

NOW CHASE TO THE CUT
We've given you all the information you need to transform your physique into the lean muscular package you've always wanted. As you take your body through this amazing transformation, keep the following bigger-picture points in mind. Don't overdiet. If you're hungry, feed your body the proper foods. If you feel weak or lousy, increase the amount of fat and protein calories you're consuming. Diet for yourself, making accommodations for your own individual needs.

Remember, this is a process, and although it can be difficult and challenging, it should be rewarding both in the doing and in the results. Good luck!

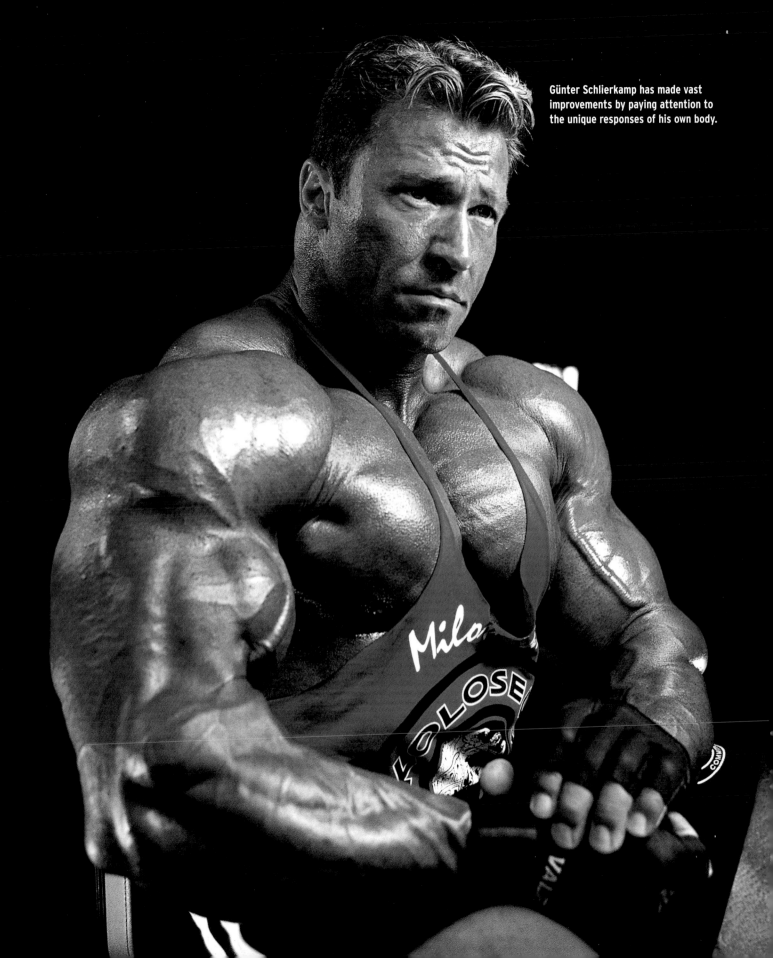

Günter Schlierkamp has made vast improvements by paying attention to the unique responses of his own body.

Now It's UP TO YOU!

Making a lifelong commitment to bodybuilding

Every pro bodybuilder will tell you that his individual quest for size has been and continues to be the greatest driving force of his life. Now that you are nearing the end of the program outlined in this book, it's time to take what you've learned and make it your own. This shift is what separates bodybuilders from guys who simply go to the gym to train with weights.

You have probably noticed how many different styles of training we recommend. These strategies included circuit training, powerlifting, bodybuilding lifting, intensity techniques and a variety of set, rep and exercise schemes. Each strategy provides your body with unique bodybuilding advantages by placing all sorts of different demands on it. By following our advice, you've learned plenty. But what to do with that knowledge? That's the question this last chapter will answer. We'll tell you how to transition off our program and onto your own. That's what ultimately makes you a bodybuilder.

WRAPPING UP THE PROGRAM

The cutting phase ("Rip It Up," Chapter 16) provides ways to maintain your muscle mass while stripping your body of fat. This is essentially the same process competitive bodybuilders go through for a competition. It's also a beneficial process for noncompetitors for a few reasons.

1. **Reducing bodyfat helps you see the muscular progress**

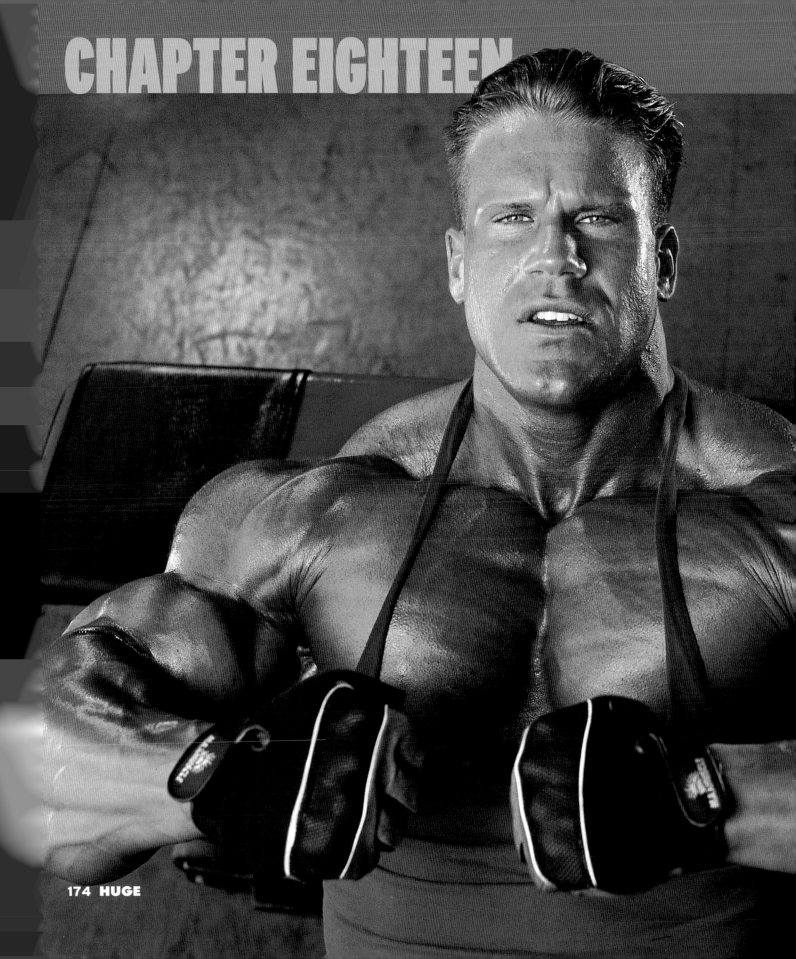

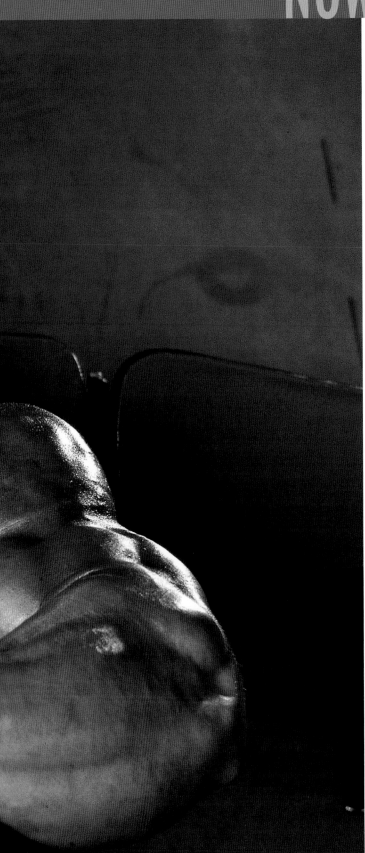

> **"Being a bodybuilder is about dedication. It's about finding what works for you, and constantly evaluating what it is you do and why you do it."**
>
> **— Jay Cutler**

you've made. When you maintain your muscles and shed fat, you create a greater shoulder-to-hip ratio. Although you lose weight, your physique appears larger and more impressive. Losing fat in your legs and midsection helps show off the detail you've added to your physique.

2. Reducing bodyfat helps create a new lower "baseline" bodyfat level. Let's say your bodyfat level was 12% before you started your diet. The process of reducing bodyfat can make you feel sluggish, weak and uninspired in the gym. As you reduced to 10% bodyfat, you probably didn't feel 100%. You may have felt even worse as your bodyfat dipped lower. However, as you transition off your diet, your bodyfat will begin to rise a little. You'll perhaps go back up to 10%, which you can easily maintain. However, now you'll feel 100% at 10% bodyfat. You'll be strong and capable of building even more muscle mass while you carry less bodyfat as your new state of normalcy. In effect, you will have reduced your baseline bodyfat from 12 to 10% while maintaining or even increasing your muscle mass. This is the ultimate goal of a bodybuilder and one of the rewards for suffering through a bodybuilding diet.

3. Stripping bodyfat helps you create the mindset of a professional bodybuilder. Many noncompetitors train hard and are able to put on plenty of muscle mass, but often their physiques don't emulate experienced bodybuilders as much as they would like. Bodyfat cycling will help you reach your fullest potential as a bodybuilder and give you that psychological edge that makes you one.

BACK TO "NORMAL" TRAINING

FLEX set up an eight-week diet for stripping bodyfat (see Chapter 17), but that's merely an average for a first-time

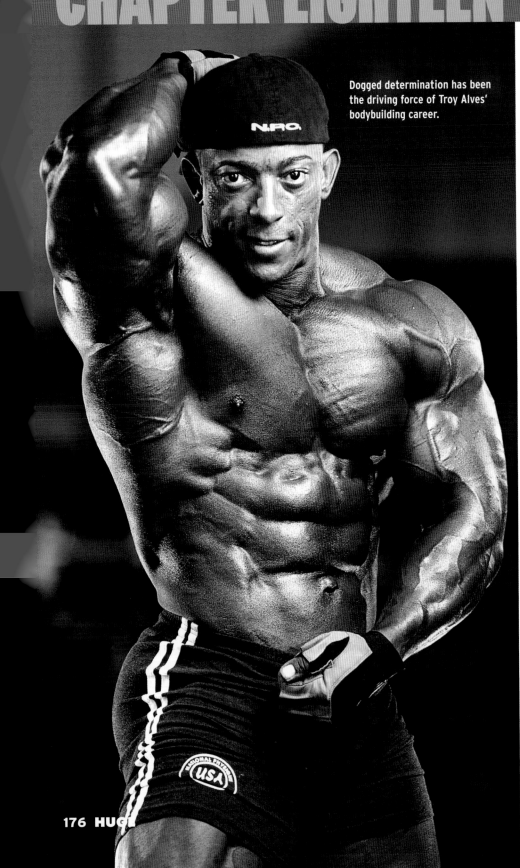

Dogged determination has been the driving force of Troy Alves' bodybuilding career.

dieter. You may feel that, after four weeks, you've shed all the bodyfat you safely can without stripping away your muscle mass. Or you may feel you need to stay on the diet an additional four weeks to get the results you seek. This is a highly individual matter, and you must trust your instincts and properly evaluate external feedback from your friends and your mirror.

When you're ready to transition off a strict bodybuilding diet, you need to plan your next move. Do you want to go through another mass-building cycle? Do you want to keep your bodyfat low as you return to a less rigorous nutrition plan? Do you need to give your body a rest from training for a week or two? Your answer is the first step in defining your own bodybuilding ambition. Once you have a clear goal, then you can begin to formulate your plan based on what you've learned from this book.

BECOMING A BODYBUILDER

It's important to understand the distinction between being a bodybuilder and being a guy who regularly goes to the gym to train with weights.

Dennis James explains his own transformation: "I started training in 1992 in Thailand. I began by going to the gym with a group of friends. I wasn't thinking about competing or getting big, but I had a bet with one guy that I could beat him lifting. Then I started putting on muscle like crazy even though I had no idea what I was doing. After three or four months, I put on so much size that people started to look at me like I was a bodybuilder."

But James said he wasn't a bodybuilder yet. "I didn't even train my legs

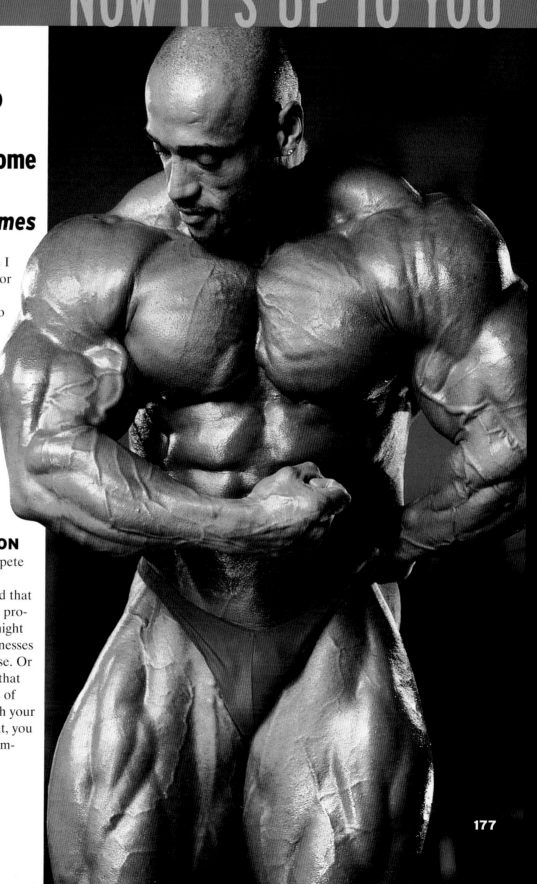

> **"Only when I made that commitment to take it to the next level did I truly become a bodybuilder."**
> **– Dennis James**

for the first couple of years because I wasn't worried about my symmetry or balance. When I finally started to think about these things, I started to focus on my weaknesses more than my strengths. I started watching bodybuilding videos and reading all the magazines. Then, I went to Gold's Gym in Venice for the first time in 1997. That inspired me to prepare to compete in my first amateur show. Only when I made that commitment to take it to the next level did I truly become a bodybuilder."

THE JOURNEY VERSUS THE DESTINATION

That doesn't mean you have to compete to be a bodybuilder. James says you become a bodybuilder when you find that one thing that causes you to make a profound commitment or sacrifice. It might be a dedication to working on weaknesses instead of strengths, as in James' case. Or it might be a dedication to the gym that takes precedence over other aspects of your life. Instead of hanging out with your friends drinking beer on Friday night, you find yourself at the gym, working hamstrings and calves.

Once you've had that epiphany,

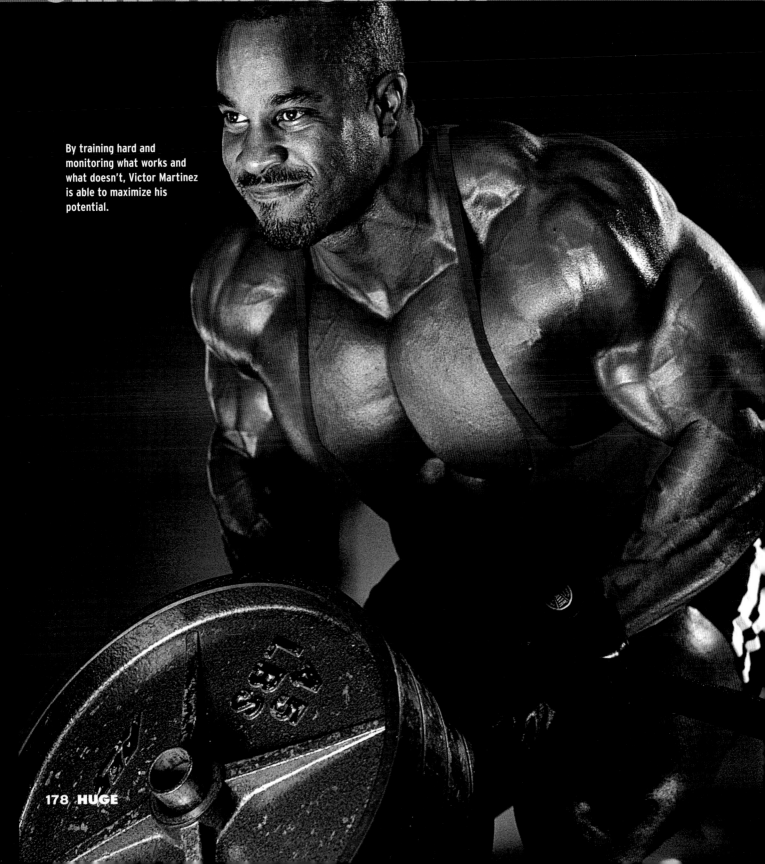

By training hard and monitoring what works and what doesn't, Victor Martinez is able to maximize his potential.

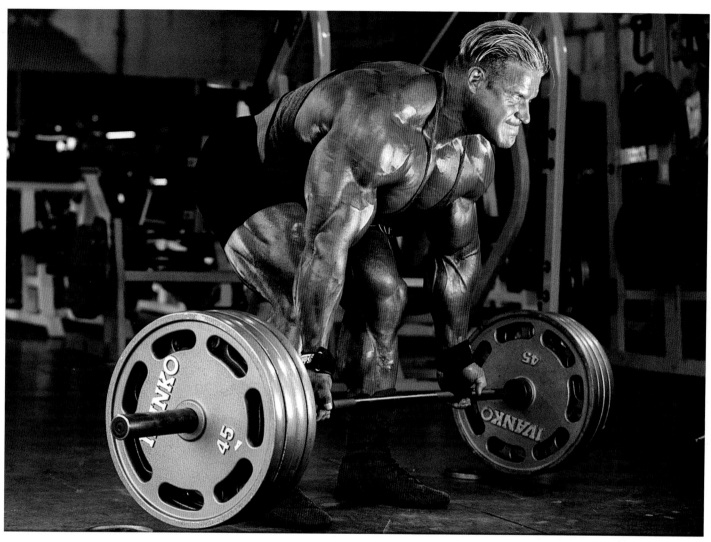

whether it occurred during the last year or whether it has yet to happen, pro bodybuilders agree that bodybuilding becomes a lifestyle, not an objective; a journey, not a destination. "If you're training for an isolated moment in time, you aren't a bodybuilder yet," Jay Cutler says. "Being a bodybuilder is about dedication. It's about finding what works for you, and constantly evaluating what it is you do and why you do it."

Cutler offers the following advice: "Keep a journal that records everything that works and doesn't work for you. Keep changing your routine every couple of months, so your body doesn't get used to your workout. Add a new

> ## "Keep a journal that records everything that works and doesn't work for you."
> ### – Jay Cutler

movement to each bodypart training every time you change your workout. But keep it simple. Don't complicate things by adding funky cable movements or too many isolation movements. Basic movements are what's going to build mass d make you a bodybuilder. If you're not cutting up for a bodybuilding show, then stick with those basic movements. Bodybuilders don't focus on how much weight they move they think about how much muscle they can build. If

you're thinking and training like a bodybuilder, you can maintain that mindset for the rest of your life. I believe I can keep going as a professional bodybuilder until I'm 45 if I keep training the way I do."

And that's the goal, ultimately. Regardless of how long Jay Cutler and Dennis James compete, you know that even after they retire, they'll still be bodybuilders. Like "Sir" or "General," "Bodybuilder" is a title that's earned. Once you achieve it, it's yours forever.

We've thrown a lot at you in this book. We hope you've realized it's more than a clever title and a big concept: This book is the culmination of decades of in-the-trenches experience and scientific analysis by the *FLEX* brain trust.

If you've followed the program in this book for a year, the question now is: What plan do you follow for the next year and the year after that? The truth is, for a bodybuilder, the journey never ends. Over the next 12 months, you may want to go back and repeat the program phase for phase, or you may want to concentrate for an extended period on a specific segment. The path toward fulfilling the limits of your own physical potential is an individual one, and one best plotted by you.

Whatever gains in muscular size you have made from our program, the greatest gain should be the self-knowledge you've reaped regarding how your body responded to the nuances of this 12-month program. You may have responded spectacularly to some aspects, while other elements may not have worked for you at all. If something worked for you, exploit it; if something didn't work, discard it. Learn from those experiences, and use them as points of reference to determine your future strategy as you transition into becoming the expert on the means to develop your physique to its fullest capacity. Keep pushing, keep experimenting and adapting — above all, keep learning — and you will never stop progressing.

This book represents a solid launching pad for you to lift off and further explore the potential of your inner space. You are now ready to take on the mantle of becoming the master of your own physique destiny. Bon voyage, and as you take the next step in your lifelong size odyssey, *FLEX* will continue to leave the light on for you. **FLEX**

nal analysis, if you become a champion nie Coleman, you become an expert elf.